NO-RISK
Pilates

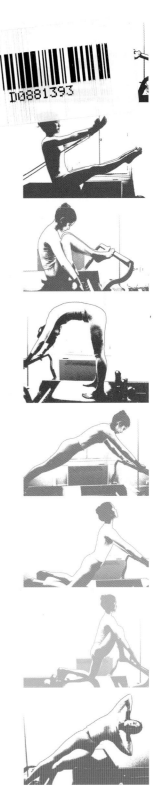

NO-RISK
Pilates

8 Techniques
for a Safe
Full-Body Workout

Blandine Calais-Germain
and **Bertrand Raison**

Translated by Martine Curtis-Oakes

Healing Arts Press
Rochester, Vermont • Toronto, Canada

BOCA RATON PUBLIC LIBRARY
BOCA RATON, FLORIDA

Healing Arts Press
One Park Street
Rochester, Vermont 05767
www.HealingArtsPress.com

Healing Arts Press is a division of Inner Traditions International

Copyright © 2010 by Éditions Désiris
English translation copyright © 2012 by Inner Traditions International

Originally published in French under the title *Pilates sans risque: 8 risques du Pilates et comment les ÉVITER*
First U.S. edition published in 2012 by Healing Arts Press

All rights reserved. No part of this book may be reproduced or utilized in any form or by any means, electronic or mechanical, including photocopying, recording, or by any information storage and retrieval system, without permission in writing from the publisher.

Note to the reader: This book is intended as an informational guide. The remedies, approaches, and techniques described herein are meant to supplement, and not to be a substitute for, professional medical care or treatment. They should not be used to treat a serious ailment without prior consultation with a qualified health care professional.

Library of Congress Cataloging-in-Publication Data
Calais-Germain, Blandine.
  [Pilates sans risque. English]
  No-risk pilates : 8 techniques for a safe full-body workout / Blandine Calais-Germain and Bertrand Raison ; translated by Martine Curtis-Oakes. — 1st U.S. ed.
      p. cm.
  Translated from French.
  Includes bibliographical references and index.
  Summary: "An illustrated, anatomical guide to improve the benefits of your Pilates workout while also preventing injury"—Provided by publisher.
  ISBN 978-1-59477-443-0 (pbk.) — ISBN 978-1-59477-697-7 (e-book)
  1. Pilates method. I. Raison, Bertrand. II. Title.
  RA781.4.C35 2012
  613.7192—dc23

                                                              2011048234

Printed and bound in China by Oceanic Graphic International, Inc.

10 9 8 7 6 5 4 3 2 1

Drawings by Blandine Calais-Germain

Text design and layout by Virginia Scott Bowman
This book was typeset in Garamond Premier Pro and Gill Sans with Helvetica and Gill Sans used as display typefaces

For further information about Blandine Calais-Germain's work go to **www.calais-germain.com**.

✦ ✦ ✦

This book is dedicated to Jerome Andrews, an American in Paris, who, taught by Joseph Pilates, was one of the first teachers of the Pilates method in France. A choreographer and dancer, he had a passion for making his students want to move their "carcass."

CONTENTS

ACKNOWLEDGMENTS

The authors would like to thank those who helped with or supported the creation of this work.

Thanks to Martine Curtis-Oakes, owner of A-Lyne Centre de Formation, Paris, France, for all of the fruitful exchanges of information.

Thanks to Simone Ushirobira, who was willing to perform the exercises over and over again during the photo shoots.

Thanks to Françoise Contreras, Brigitte Hap, and Alison Liddiart, for their gracious presence.

Thanks to Florence, for her watchful eye and wisdom.

Thanks to the numerous people who requested this information during Anatomy of Movement workshops, whose questions guided us in the organization of this book.

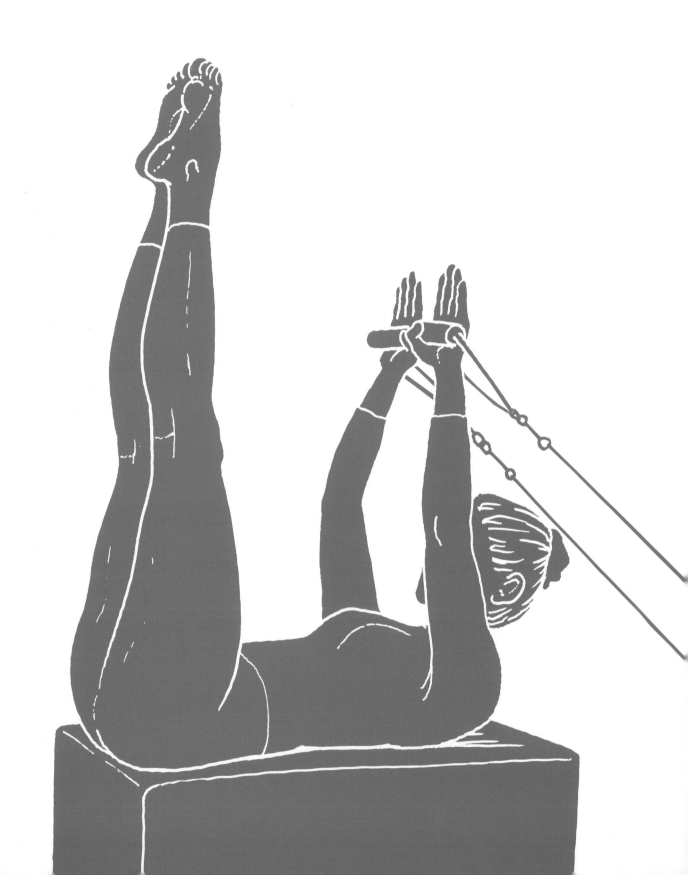

INTRODUCTION

The purpose of this book is to show the anatomical effects of Pilates exercises, specifically of exercises on the Reformer. Using eight exercises as a starting point, *No-Risk Pilates* explores the logic of each movement and some potential adverse effects. Each chapter examines a specific risk, looks at why it occurs, and proposes solutions. Finally, we look at similar Pilates Reformer and mat exercises that pose the same concerns. With each example, the practice is linked to a particular joint, such as the pelvis or femur, an area of the body like the perineum, or structures like the ligaments of the spine.

While each chapter focuses on a particular Pilates movement, along with its primary associated potential problem, this is not to say that this is the only problem that could possibly arise with this movement, or that we encounter this problem only when making this specific movement. On the contrary, many of the problems that we will examine coincide in one movement, and of course we encounter these problems in many movements outside of the realm of Pilates. The presentation is intended to serve an as an example that you can use to analyze other movement experiences.

The eight chapters are designed to provide the reader with a straightforward way to understand the concepts, by linking practical application with associated anatomical considerations.

How to Use this Book

No-Risk Pilates has several levels of content:

+ text written in straightforward language;
+ numerous illustrations and their captions; and
+ boxed areas with additional explanatory information.

Each chapter is devoted to a specific Reformer exercise and contains:

+ a description of the movement (under the heading Principles of the Exercise);
+ a breakdown of the anatomy involved in the exercise (Anatomical Landmarks);
+ a discussion of the risks that certain parts of the exercise can create (Consequences);
+ suggested solutions and methods of prevention (Solutions and Prevention); and
+ identification of other movements on the Reformer and mat that carry the same risks as the highlighted exercise (Other Exercises).

Terminology

While *No-Risk Pilates* assumes some basic knowledge of Pilates vocabulary, the book was written for anyone who wants to deepen their Pilates practice and their understanding of the method; it is not intended for the exclusive use of those in the medical or paramedical professions. For this reason, terms and nomenclature are often taken from common usage, rather than from standard scientific forms.

Certain terms used in this book have intentionally been chosen so as to remain accessible. For example, the word *leg* is often used to indicate the entire limb. Expressions such as *lie down on your back* or *lie down on your side* have been chosen over *dorsal* (or *lateral*) *decubitus*. International anatomical nomenclature has been preserved when it's accessible. When it's not, we've chosen to use the word that is in current usage in a particular country. For example, *cubitus,* which is common in French terminology, has been replaced by *ulna* in this English edition.

About Joseph Pilates

At the beginning of the twentieth century, Joseph Hubertus Pilates (1883–1967) was instrumental in a revolution that turned ideas about movement upside down. Born near Dusseldorf, the young Pilates, who suffered from asthma and rickets, became obsessed with transforming himself into an athlete. While working in a brewery, he pursued multiple physical disciplines. He was no doubt encouraged in these disciplines by his parents, who managed a gym. In 1912 he went to England to continue his training as a boxer, and he was hired there, along with his brother, to perform in a circus.

At the beginning of World War I, however, Pilates was interned on the Isle of Man along with other German nationals. Here he began helping his less fortunate companions, particularly the sick and injured. At that time, it was forbidden for patients to leave their beds, but Joseph found a way to help them exercise anyway: he equipped the beds with springs and straps, creating the predecessor of the Trap Table (also called the Cadillac). With this apparatus, the bedridden patients could begin to move their arms and legs against resistance, thereby reaping the physical and psychological rewards of movement. His regimen proved to be very successful, and its early adopters enjoyed a speedier recovery than those around them.

At the end of the war Pilates returned to Germany, where he continued his exploration of movement reeducation. He trained athletes, the military, and the police, while continuing to refine his equipment. He developed the apparatus as a means of creating conditions that would encourage specific muscles to respond. Resistance from the apparatus could stimulate deep-muscle engagement and promote concentration: the whole body was involved.

The political climate was changing in

Germany, and Pilates emigrated to the United States around 1925. There, he met his wife, Clara, and the two opened a studio on New York City's Eighth Avenue. Dancers from the New York City Ballet and Martha Graham came to work with them, along with people from all walks of life. But it wasn't until the 1970s and '80s that media attention brought the Pilates method to the mainstream. Today, from Australia to Brazil to Europe, the number of people who practice Pilates is in the millions.

The Reformer

Among the numerous machines or "apparatus" invented by Joseph Pilates, the Reformer, along with the Trap Table and the Chair, hold the most prominent positions. Exercises on these apparatus, as well as on the mat, form the basis of the Pilates method. The Reformer is probably the most internationally recognizable of all the apparatus. It was known in France between the 1950s and '80s as simply "the machine"— a bit different from its American counterpart, but in principle the same.

Basic Form
The Reformer is composed of a rectangular frame in which a sliding carriage moves. Most Reformer exercises are done while lying on the back, although there are also exercises done on the knees, in a seated position, or standing.

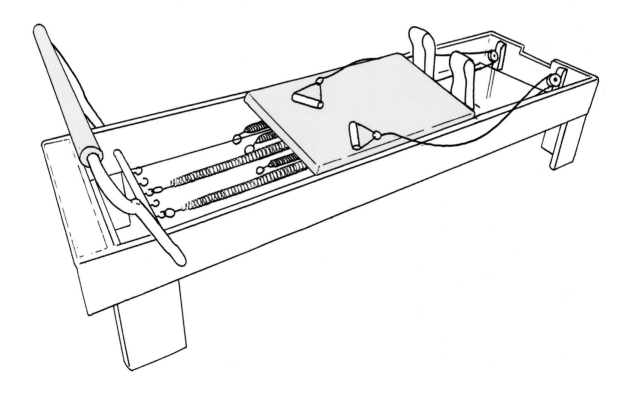

Other accessories can be added. The repertoire includes hundreds of combinations and a rich vocabulary of variations.

Bar and Springs

At the front end of the Reformer is a bar that is adjustable in height, and on some models it can be moved along the length of the Reformer frame. In a lying position, the feet can be placed on this bar; in a kneeling position, the hands will be placed on it. Underneath this bar are springs, which connect the moving carriage to another bar fixed to the frame. The springs are of different resistance, and the number of springs varies with the Reformer model. Their usefulness lies in the ability to provide the user with resistance during pushing and pulling of the carriage.

The Carriage

This moveable bed has two immobile shoulder rests at its far end that assume different functions. Depending on the user's position and the exercise being performed, these shoulder rests can be alternately used as support for the shoulders, the feet, or the hands. Between the two shoulder rests is a head rest that can be raised or lowered and can also accommodate pressure from different parts of the body depending on the exercise. Sometimes a box about sixteen inches high is placed on the carriage for exercises in which the user needs to be elevated, as in the Teaser and Side Sit-ups (see pages 17 and 94).

Finally, parallel to the springs there is a second system designed to move the carriage. Two cords fixed on the back edges of both sides of the carriage run through pulleys attached to the back of the frame. The cords loop back to the carriage, where they terminate in loops or handles. Therefore, without pushing on the bar, you can move the carriage by placing the hands or feet in the loops and pulling.

1

FOOTWORK

and Yo-yoing of the Pelvis

When executed poorly, the Footwork exercise causes repeated rocking of the pelvis, which has an impact on the intervertebral disks.

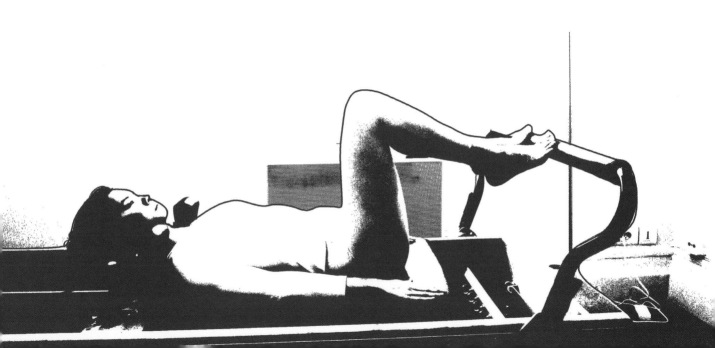

Principles of the Exercise

Starting Position

Lie on the carriage with the shoulders against the shoulder rests, the legs and feet parallel and a bit separated, the toes on the bar, and the knees flexed.

> "Pilates position," which is different from the position you see here, requires a slight external rotation of the legs. It's desirable to alternate the positions (parallel and turned-out) in order to change the muscular engagement.

The Movement

This series progresses through different foot positions, with the arches and heels on the bar. Comparable to a *plié* in dance, the exercise engages the same three joints: the hips, the knees, and the ankles.

Extension of all three of these joints is required to push the carriage out, while flexion of the three joints is necessary to bring the carriage back in. During the return, the feet must maintain their force against the bar to resist the action of the springs.

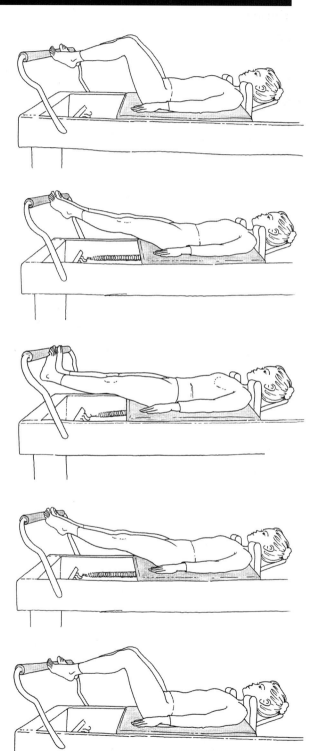

Observations

During the course of this exercise, the pelvis has a tendency to rock to the front and back in relation to the trunk (see box). This rocking is especially pronounced in the Tendon Stretch—the third Footwork variation depicted, which accentuates the forward tipping of the pelvis. Why?

Because the extension of the hips, knees, and ankles together tends to antevert the pelvis, while flexion of these three joints together tends to retrovert the pelvis. We therefore end up "scissoring" the pelvis back and forth repeatedly.

What we mean when we say that the pelvis "tips" forward or backward is that the pelvis moves in relation to a determined point of reference—the position wherein the iliac crests are perpendicular to the carriage and the ischia (sitz bones) aren't touching the carriage. In this position the physiological curves of the spine are respected.

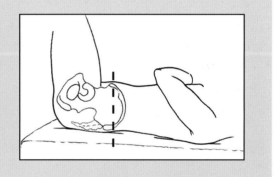

Anatomical Landmarks

Extending the Legs Causes Anteversion of the Pelvis

Initially, we tend to use the pressure of the pelvis rather than the pressure of the feet against the bar. This causes us to flatten the lumbar spine against the carriage and bring the iliac spines toward the carriage—i.e., retroversion.

Then, when we start extending the legs, the opposite happens: the iliac spines move forward and the pelvis goes into anteversion, accentuating the lumbar curve. Why?

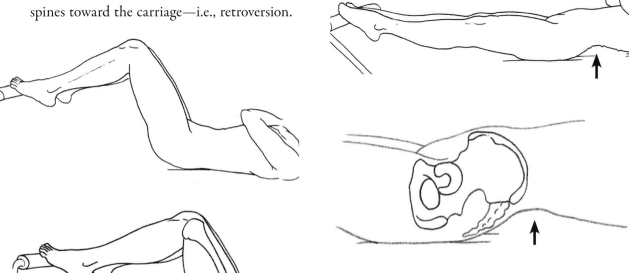

> *Anteversion* is the tilting of the iliac crests forward—toward the ceiling if you're on your back. Anteversion increases the lumbar curve.

The Ligaments at the Front of the Hip Pull the Iliac Crests Forward

Both the ligaments and the primary hip flexors—the psoas, iliacus, sartorius, rectus femoris, and tensor fascia latae—are put progressively under tension during the push-out phase of this exercise. When these ligaments and muscles are put under tension, they pull the iliac crests forward and the pelvis goes into anteversion. Dropping the heels under the bar increases the anteversion.

> With the exception of the psoas, the primary hip flexors attach at the front of the iliac bone and are located on the anterior surface of the pelvis and the thigh. The psoas insertions are situated along the lumbar vertebrae. That said, stretching the psoas increases the curve of the lumbar spine and favors anteversion.

The Return: Leg Flexion Encourages Pelvic Retroversion

During the return movement, flexion of the hip increases, and the pelvis tends to roll the iliac spines backward; in other words, the pelvis goes into retroversion. Why?

> *Retroversion* is the tilting of the iliac crests backward, which flattens the lumbar curve.

The Posterior Muscles of the Thigh Pull the Iliac Crests Backward

This time, it is not the anterior muscles of the thigh that are pulled, but the posterior muscles. Under tension, these muscles pull the iliac crests backward. The iliac spines move toward the carriage and the ischia move away from the carriage, reversing the anteversion. If the flexion goes beyond 90°, the pelvis is placed in retroversion.

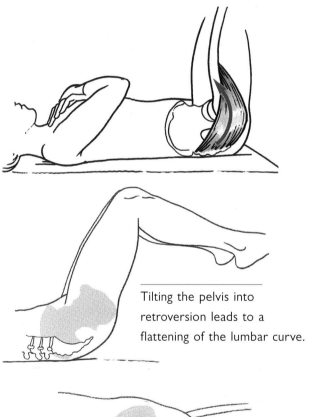

Tilting the pelvis into retroversion leads to a flattening of the lumbar curve.

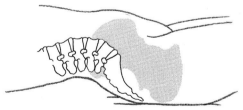

Tilting the pelvis into anteversion leads to an increase in the lumbar curve.

Consequences

The Yo-yo Effect

Flexion of the legs/anteversion brings the anterior surfaces of the vertebrae closer together: the front of the disk is squeezed and the back of the disk is stretched.

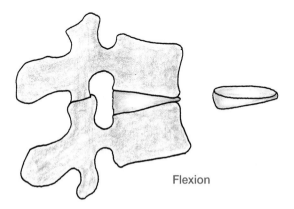

Flexion

Extension of the legs/retroversion brings the posterior surfaces of the vertebrae closer together: the back of the disk is pinched while the front is stretched.

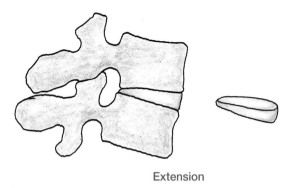

Extension

This back-and-forth play between retroversion and anteversion can cause "scissoring" of the lower intervertebral disks.

The intervertebral disks are very small cushions made up of fibrocartilage. They are interposed between the anterior parts of the vertebrae, known as the vertebral bodies, and they allow for movement of the spine in all directions. They also serve as shock absorbers for the spine.

Each disk is composed of a fibrous ring—the annulus—that resembles the layers of an onion. The annulus encircles the gelatinous nucleus housed in the center.

These two components should remain stable for proper functioning of the disk. However, when the disk is damaged, fissures can form in the annulus and the nucleus can become unstable.

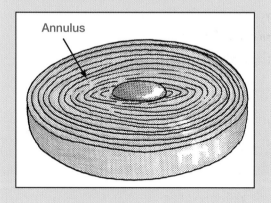

Annulus

Why Is This Rocking a Risk Factor?

Lumbar flexion and extension are not harmful in and of themselves. However, the yo-yoing movement from one to the other tends to be too dramatic and can cause the posterior and anterior parts of the annulus to be too pinched and too stretched.

At the same time that the yo-yo effect is being produced, there is strong compression of the disk, in part due to the resistance of the springs. These factors combine to over-work the disk, especially the annulus, which is repeatedly "scissored."

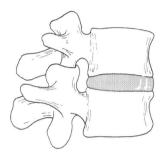

L5/S1: A Vulnerable Area

Among the lower intervertebral disks, the yo-yo effect has the greatest impact on L5/S1, situated between the top of the sacrum and the fifth lumbar vertebra.

> The sacrum is the most posterior bone of the pelvis. Its lower end is joined to the coccyx, which is the lowest part of the vertebral column and is composed of five fused vertebrae. This area is easy to locate on yourself because it is convex and fits easily into your cupped hand.

This is the lowest disk; in the spinal column; therefore it's the one that receives the most "load," and is often overworked and fragile.

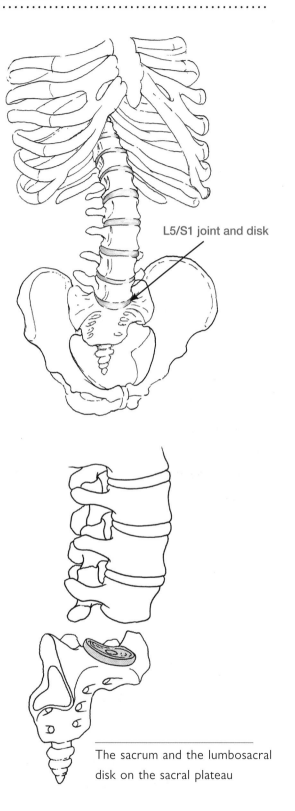

L5/S1 joint and disk

The sacrum and the lumbosacral disk on the sacral plateau

Solutions and Prevention

How to Stabilize the Pelvis During the Push-Out

We can prevent anteversion of the pelvis—and thereby prevent yo-yoing—by stabilizing it during the exercise.

1. Identify the Moment When the Pelvis Starts to Tip Forward

Repeat the exercise on the Reformer or on the mat. Starting with the pelvis in a neutral position and the knees a little bent, extend the legs out (glide the feet on the mat).

Notice when the pelvis starts to antevert.*

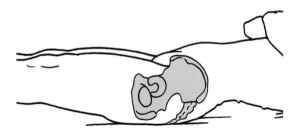

2. Use the Abdominal Muscles to Counteract Anteversion

Once we've identified the moment of anteversion, we can stabilize the pelvis with the abdominal muscles, specifically, the rectus abdominus. It's this muscle that pulls the pelvis into retroversion and can therefore prevent it from moving in the opposite direction.

---

*For more information on identifying pelvic anteversion, see page 75 of *No-Risk Abs*, by Blandine Calais-Germain (Rochester, Vt.: Healing Arts Press, 2011).

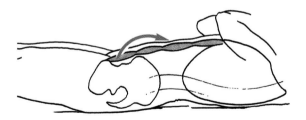

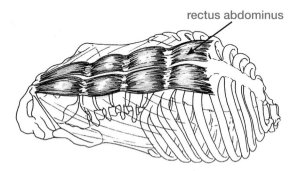

rectus abdominus

Finding the moment of anteversion in advance allows us to recruit the rectus abdominus at that moment and then regulate the amount of contraction needed throughout the exercise.

How to Stabilize the Pelvis on the Return

The pelvis can be kept in a neutral position on the return in order to avoid retroversion.

1. Identify the Moment When the Pelvis Tilts Backward

Try the exercise on the Reformer or on the mat without the bar and with your knees flexed.

Starting from a neutral pelvic position, draw the knees progressively toward the sternum. Notice the moment that the pelvis starts tilting backward into retroversion. It's this tilting that we need to prevent.

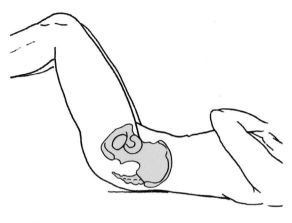

2. Counteract Retroversion of the Pelvis

Once we've determined when the pelvis starts to retrovert, we can control it by recruiting the dorsal muscles—multifidus, interspinalis, longissimus, iliocostalis, and latissimus dorsi. These dorsal muscles are situated at the back of the trunk, along the spine, and along the ribs. They all oppose the action of the abdominals, and most of them bring the pelvis into anteversion.

Alternating the action of the abdominals and the dorsals is a good way to control the position of the pelvis. Tracking exactly when the pelvis begins to tilt in either direction allows us to activate these muscle groups to keep the pelvis stable and above all to protect L5/S1. To control the movement of the pelvis even more, we can place a small cushion under the lumbar curve, which can help us to sense when the pelvis is stable. However, be careful not to crush or lift away from the cushion.

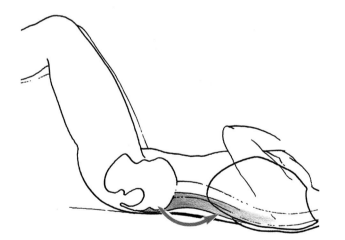

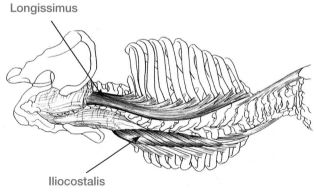

Longissimus

Iliocostalis

Other Exercises That Risk Yo-yoing the Pelvis

Reformer Exercises

There are several Reformer exercises that can destabilize the pelvis and lead to yo-yoing.

Hundred

During this exercise, be careful not to press your lower back into the carriage while trying to hold your legs in position. Also make sure that you don't increase the lumbar curve when your legs are lowered.

Coordination

This exercise is a variation of the Hundred, and we find the same problems of pelvic instability.

Frog and Leg Circles

Follow the same precautions as in the previous exercises.

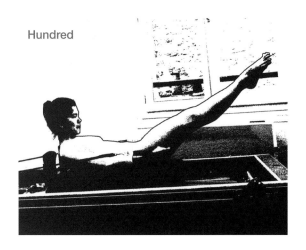

Hundred

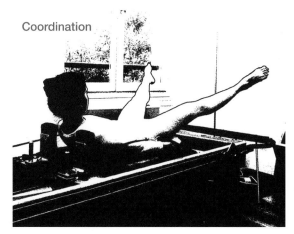

Coordination

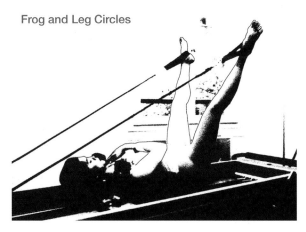

Frog and Leg Circles

Side Split

This is a lateral split, and we need to prevent the pelvis from moving toward either the front or the back. As in Footwork, when we push the carriage out, the pelvis tends to antevert, while on the return it tends to retrovert.

Long Stretch

Stabilize the pelvis throughout the whole exercise. The play between the abdominals and the dorsals is essential for keeping the heel-pelvis-shoulder alignment.

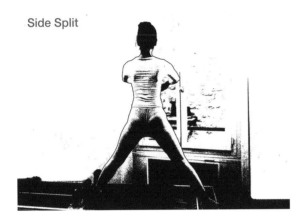

Side Split

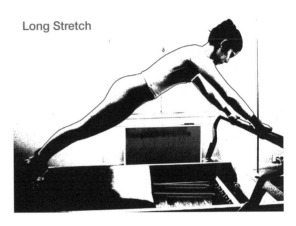

Long Stretch

Mat Exercises

The mat exercises that carry the risk of yo-yoing the pelvis include the following.

Hundred

This exercise is almost identical to the one performed on the Reformer. On the mat, however, the lack of springs reduces pressure on the lumbar area, and therefore reduces the risk of the yo-yoing.

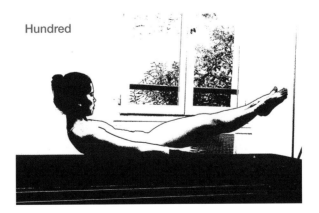

Hundred

Single Leg Circle, Single Leg Stretch, Double Leg Stretch, Scissors, Crisscross, Double Leg Lower Lifts

Single Leg Circles, along with all of the exercises that follow—collectively called the "stomach series"—carry the same risk of pelvic instability and therefore the risk of weakening the lumbar disks.

Corkscrew

Turning the legs around the axis of the pelvis is a direct test of pelvic stability. Each time that the legs are moved away from and toward the pelvis, this instability is augmented.

Side Kick Series Front and Back, Bicycle, Rond de Jambe

This series specifically emphasizes the need for pelvic stability so that the pelvis doesn't move forward when the leg goes to the front, and doesn't rock backward when the leg goes to the back. This is an excellent opportunity to apply the principle of abdominal-dorsal engagement to prevent the yo-yo effect.

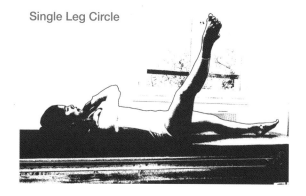

Single Leg Circle

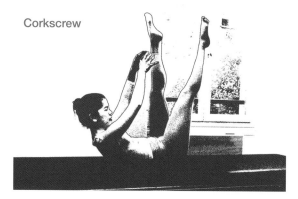

Corkscrew

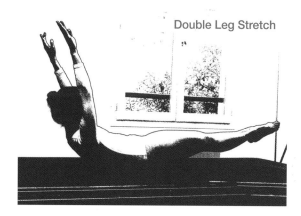

Double Leg Stretch

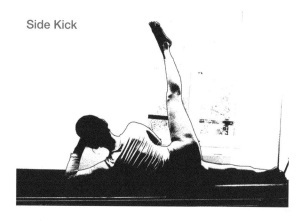

Side Kick

2
TEASER

and Its Effect on the Perineum

The Teaser exercise involves a rolling up of the spine, which, when poorly executed, can cause unwanted pressure on the lower pelvis and the perineum.

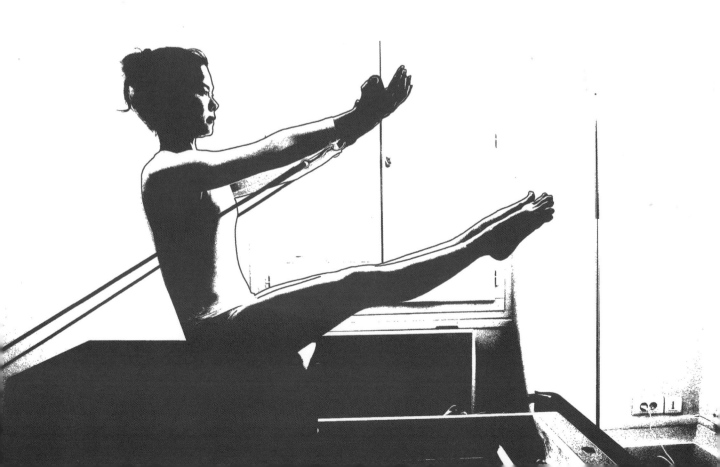

Principles of the Exercise

Starting Position

Lie down on your back on the long box, with your feet on the bar and your arms at your sides, with your hands in the handles or loops. In this position, your trunk will be higher than your limbs. With the arms positioned behind the trunk and the hips extended (here, stretching the hip flexors), the spine is taken into extension and this causes the pelvis to antevert.

The Movement

The Teaser consists of two steps—the push-out and the return. On the push-out, the upper part of the spine is flexed and then the whole trunk is lifted off the box and into an oblique position, with the weight behind the sitz bones.

At the same time, the hips flex while the legs remain straight and the hands press into the handles and move forward and up with the elbows straight.

On the return, the same movements are executed in the reverse order, except that the spine starts by flexing to place the vertebrae down sequentially on the box.*

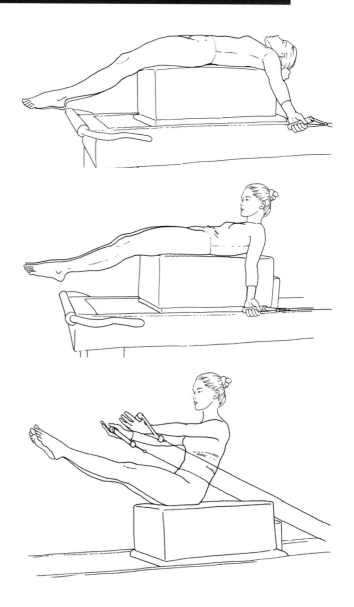

***

*This exercise also calls for the lowering and lifting of the legs once you are in the seated "Teaser" position. As we have already seen in chapter 1, the lowering and lifting of the legs can cause yo-yoing of the pelvis.

Observations

We often notice that in the course of this exercise the abdomen tends to bulge. What happens when the upper part of the trunk moves toward the lower part?

Spinal Flexion Engages the Abdominal Muscles

Flexion begins as the head lifts (1), which is accomplished by the contraction of the neck flexors.

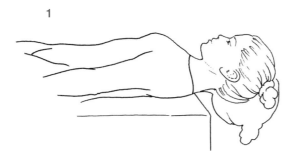

Then the shoulders join the head and neck in flexion (2), thanks to the action of the pectoral muscles.

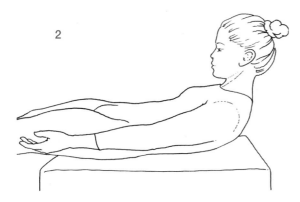

During these first two steps, the abdominals act to fix the rib cage to the pelvis. In this action they work statically, or isometrically, meaning that they don't move the skeleton. This is not to say that the contraction is not intense; it can become quite intense once the shoulders are lifted.

> We call a muscle contraction *static* or *isometric* when it does not bring the points of insertion closer together. In the example of the abdominal muscles, a static contraction stabilizes the pelvis and the ribs—the two areas where the abdominals insert—without bringing them toward each other.

Next comes flexion of the upper thoracic spine (3). Because this area is not extremely mobile, the mid-thoracic area quickly joins in, facilitated by a shortening of the abdominal muscles. This shortening decreases the length of the anterior trunk and compresses the abdominal space.

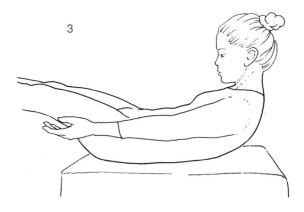

Lowering the Ribs

When we flex the spine, the rib cage moves at the same time. When the rib cage drops, it puts pressure on the lower abdomen and the perineum.

When we flex the neck (1), the first rib lowers. As we lift the shoulder blades (2), the upper ribs drop. The abdominals, which are the muscles that lower the ribs, contribute to the complete dropping of the thoracic rib cage (3).

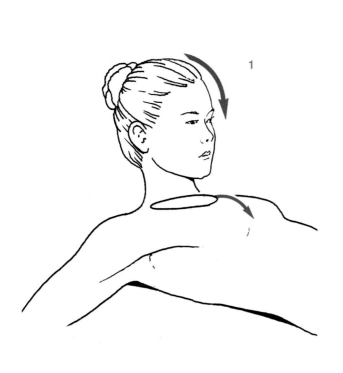

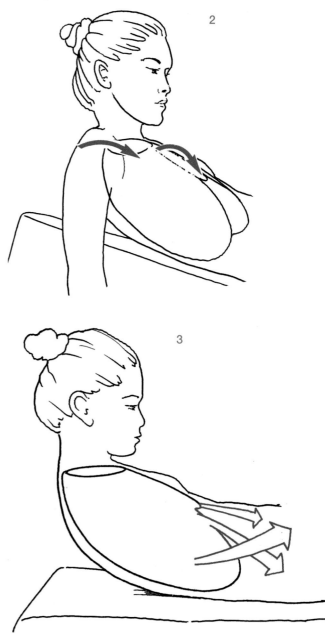

Consequences

Rolling Up from the Head Pushes the Abdominal Mass Downward

The belly, or rather the abdominal wall, contains the viscera. This mass can be compared to a bowl of liquid. While its mass can't be compressed, nor its volume changed, what does change is its form. The form of the abdomen changes depending on how the trunk moves.*

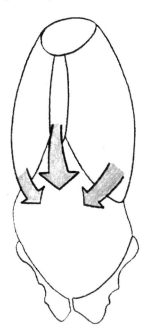

When the Abdominal Mass Moves Downward, the Belly Bulges

Rolling the spine toward the pelvis pushes the viscera in the same direction and they move

---

*For more information on how the abdominal muscles affect the viscera, see pages 18 and 21 of Blandine Calais-Germain's *No-Risk Abs*.

lower in the abdomen: in the course of this exercise we notice that the abdomen often tends to bulge from the effort of the abdominals and pressure from the rib cage.

The effects of this pressure are exacerbated if we try to "help" ourselves during the toughest part of the roll-up with a forceful exhalation when the shoulder blades leave the mat. Similarly, a diaphragmatic inhalation, which pushes the belly toward the pelvis, also causes the belly to bulge.

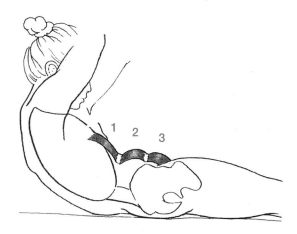

Four Factors That Contribute to Belly Bulging during the Teaser

+ Rolling the spine up
+ Dropping the ribs
+ The "descending" contraction of the abdominals, which reinforces the head-to-pelvis movement and pushes the abdomen even lower
+ The exhalation that tends to close the ribs

When the Abdominal Mass Moves Downward, It Puts Pressure on the Perineum

The interior of the pelvis can be visualized as a funnel made up of two parts, one superimposed on the other. The upper portion, the largest, is the *greater pelvis*. The lower and narrower part is the *lesser pelvis*. It's in this lower part that the perineum is situated, at the lowest level of the lesser pelvis and therefore at the lowest level of the trunk.*

This area is composed of a variety of structures: skin, muscle, viscera (bladder, rectum, the prostate in men, and the vagina and uterus in women). The muscles take the shape of a hammock, forming the pelvic floor that supports the viscera.

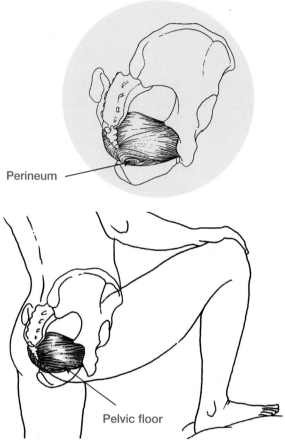

Perineum

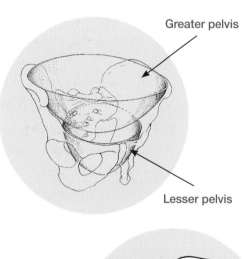

Greater pelvis

Lesser pelvis

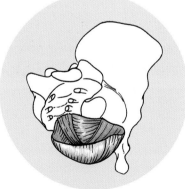

Pelvic floor

Because the perineum is situated at the base of the pelvis, it receives the constant pressure of the viscera. Because the Teaser exercise pushes the visceral mass toward the pelvis, it puts additional pressure on the area. This repeated excessive pressure on the perineum can encourage incontinence, prolapse in women, or compression of the prostate in men.

*See *The Female Pelvis: Anatomy & Exercises,* by Blandine Calais-Germain (Seattle: Eastland Press, 2003).

Solutions and Prevention

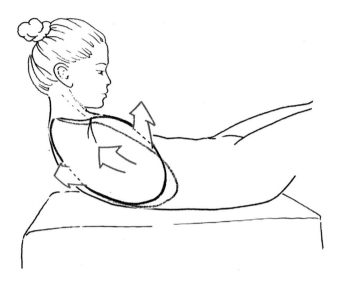

How to Lighten the Pressure on the Perineum

There are a number of things we can do to reduce pressure on the perineum during the Teaser exercise.

1. Open the Ribs to Encourage the Belly to Lift

Try the Teaser again on the Reformer or on the mat. Start with the pelvis in a neutral position, knees a little bent, then lengthen the legs. (If you're on the mat, glide the feet along the floor.)

The lowering of the thoracic rib cage pushes the viscera toward the belly, so we're trying to achieve the opposite by opening the ribs during the entire roll-up. When we open the ribs, the thorax acts like a suction cup and pulls the viscera up from the abdomen. The belly lifts and flattens.

2. Use the Arms

Take care not to lower the arms too much when you're balancing in the seated position. Keep them as high as possible, as this tends to open the thorax.

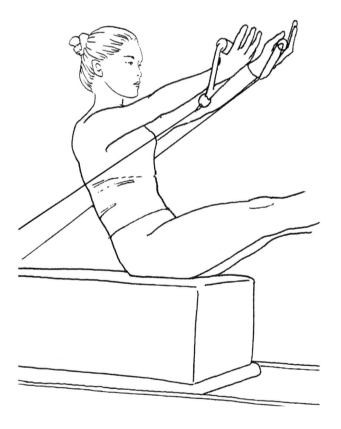

3. Use the Abdominal Muscles
to Lift the Belly

The abdominal muscles can be employed to lift the belly, if they're used properly. Instead of activating them from the top to the bottom, it's possible to contract them from the bottom to the top, which will push the abdominal mass upward.

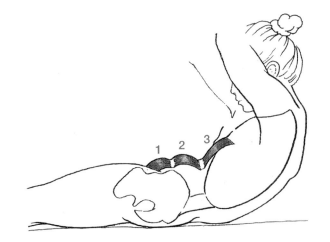

4. Inhale When Initiating the Teaser

The Teaser usually begins on an exhalation, which has the consequence of pushing the viscera in the direction of the lesser pelvis. This intensifies the downward pressure, which is then increased by the act of rolling the spine up.

We can choose to do the opposite and inhale on the roll-up, which will open the ribs. This will augment the upward draw from the thorax and reduce the pressure on the perineum.

5. Keep the Waist Lifted

To reduce the downward push on the viscera, we can keep the waist long. This is an area that the weight of the rib cage tends to shorten. We should work to increase the space between the ribs and the pelvis when doing this exercise, since it will tend to collapse naturally under our own body weight and the pull of gravity.

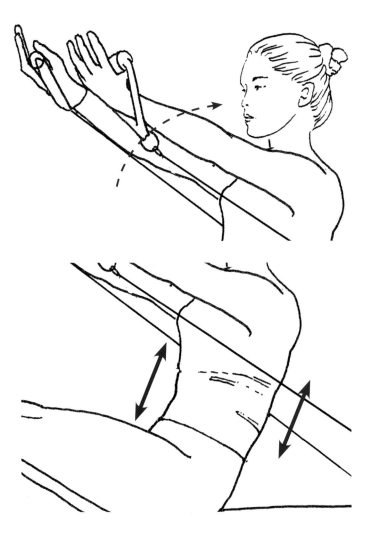

Other Exercises That Carry Similar Risks for the Perineum

Reformer Exercises

As a general rule, spinal flexion from the head pushes the belly toward the perineum, so any exercises that flex the spine will have a tendency to put too much pressure there.

Stomach Massage

One of the positions in this series (Round Back) calls specifically for flexion of the spine and exerts strong pressure on the lesser pelvis.

Short Box Series, Round Back

This exercise is performed while seated on the box. It is a variation of the Crunch,* which is done on the mat, and has the same effect of compression on the perineum.

Elephant

Bringing the trunk toward the thighs tends to push the viscera down lower in the belly.

Stomach Massage

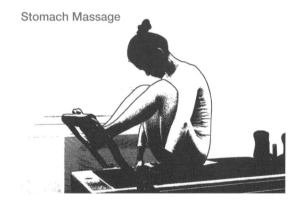

Short Box Series, Round Back

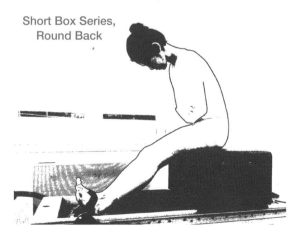

Elephant

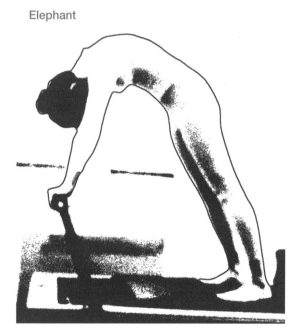

*See the analysis of this exercise in Blandine Calais-Germain's *No-Risk Abs*, pages 60–71.

Knee Stretch Round

The curling of the spine in this movement can also encourage pressure in the direction of the lesser pelvis.

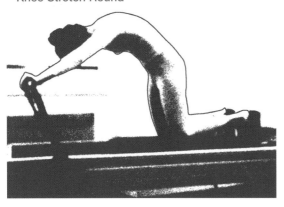

Knee Stretch Round

Rowing Series: Into the Sternum

The dynamics of this exercise are the same as with the Crunch, and have the same effect of putting pressure on the lower abdomen.

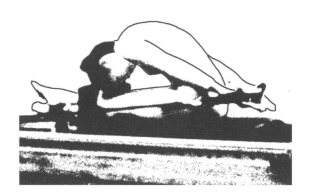

Rowing Series: Into the Sternum

Mat Exercises

Mat exercises that involve spinal flexion from the head will have the same effects on the viscera and pelvis as those on the Reformer.

In order to avoid repetition, the mat version of Teaser doesn't appear on this list. Nor does Boomerang, in which Teaser is a major component.

Roll-up (Spine Stretch Forward)

The hinge effect that brings the trunk over the thighs pushes the abdominal mass downward and thus puts pressure on the perineum.

Open-Leg Rocker

The balance required to maintain this position augments the downward pressure on the lower abdomen.

Open-Leg Rocker

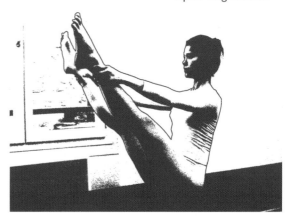

Saw

The emphasis put on bringing the trunk closer to the thigh means more weight is going to be put on the lower belly.

Seal (Rolling Like a Ball)

This rolling action, performed with the legs lifted and the trunk close to the thighs, pushes the viscera in the only direction possible—toward the perineum. This is especially true on the return.

Neck Pull

This extreme version of the Roll-up closes the angle between the trunk and the thighs, pushing the abdominal mass even lower.

Saw

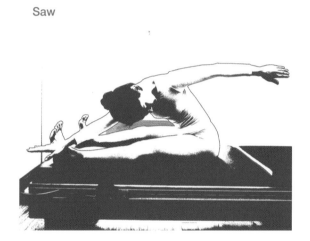

Seal (Rolling Like a Ball)

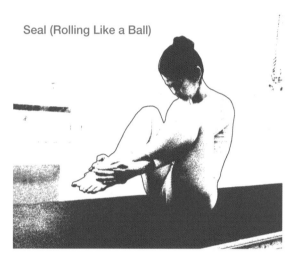

Neck Pull

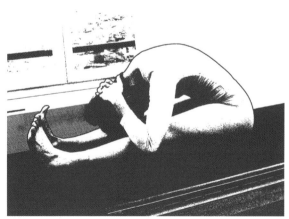

3

STOMACH MASSAGE

and Inversion of the Lumbar Curve

This exercise, done in a rounded position with the head toward the pelvis, exerts pressure—generated by the flexion—on the lower trunk. This series has several variations, but this effect is most notable in the rounded version.

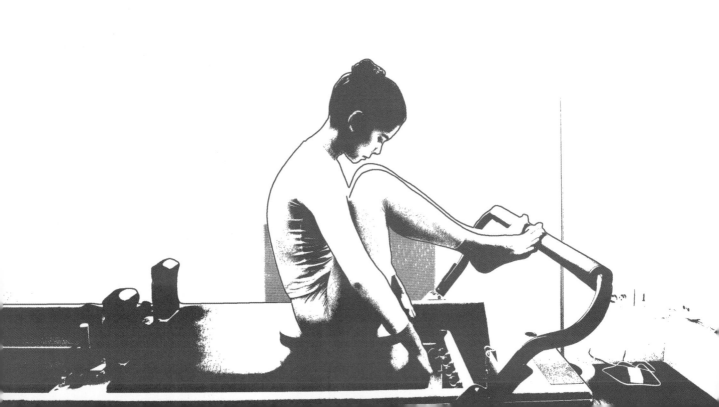

Principles of the Exercise

Starting Position

To perform this exercise, we sit on the carriage with the upper trunk slightly flexed. The fingers are at the front edge of the carriage, the legs are flexed, and the toes are on the bar.

The sequence can be done with legs either parallel or in Pilates position (with the legs in slight external rotation from the hips).

The Movement

These four movements are done in succession.

1 ✦ The feet press against the bar to extend the knees and the hips. This moves the carriage backward. The feet are pointed (ankles in plantar flexion).
2 ✦ Then, with the knees straight, the ankles flex (dorsiflexion) and the heels pass under the bar. The carriage slides forward a bit.

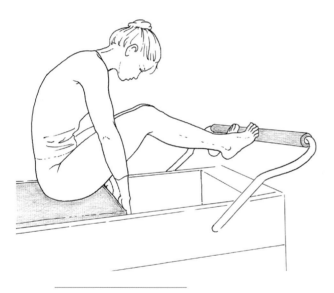

Starting position

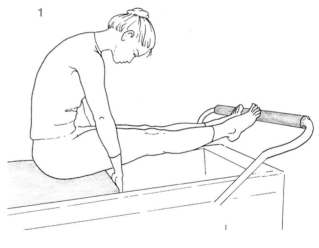

1

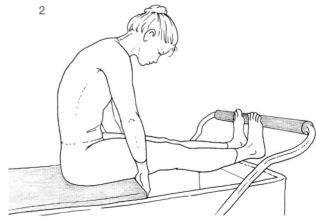

2

3 ✦ The feet are then pointed again and the carriage moves backward slightly.

4 ✦ The hips and knees flex, which brings the carriage back to starting position.

If this exercise is done correctly, the lumbar spine should be stable and able to maintain its natural curve (slightly arched).

Observations

When this exercise is being executed, or even in the starting position, the lumbar curve will often disappear. The pelvis tips into retroversion, causing flexion of the lumbar spine. Why?

Because tension in the hamstrings pulls the pelvis into retroversion.

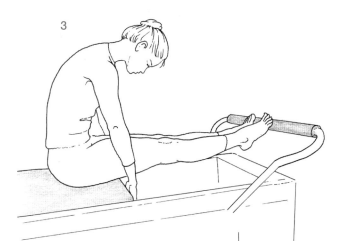

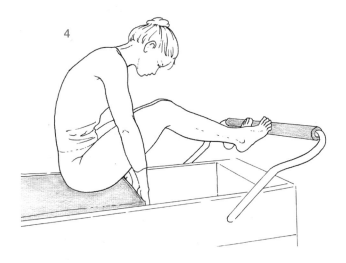

Return to starting position

Anatomical Landmarks

The Hamstrings—Masters of the Pelvis

The hamstring muscles, including semimembranosus, semitendinosus, and biceps femoris, connect the ischia (sitz bones) to the leg bones. Semimembranosus and semitendinosus connect high on the tibia, while biceps femoris connects to the head of the fibula.

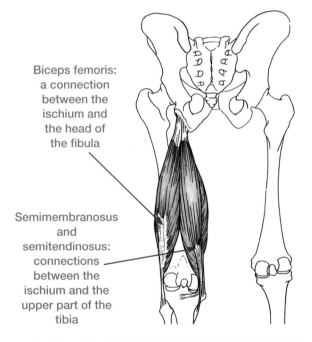

Biceps femoris: a connection between the ischium and the head of the fibula

Semimembranosus and semitendinosus: connections between the ischium and the upper part of the tibia

> The hamstrings are muscles that are often short and tight, though their length varies considerably from person to person.
>
> Beyond the hip, these muscles cross the knee. If they are tight, then they will be put under even more tension when the knee is extended. They will tend to pull on the pelvis.

Tension in the Hamstrings

If the foot is not fixed, tension in the hamstrings will act on both the hip and the knee. This will cause two inverse movements simultaneously: extension of the hip and flexion of the knee.

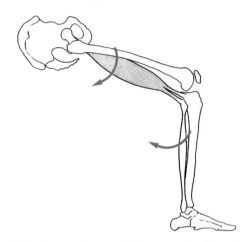

The hamstrings will be stretched by these two movements.

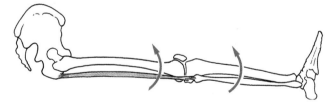

If the foot is fixed, the hamstrings become knee extensors. When the foot is in a fixed position, the hamstrings pull the tibia backward. Since the tibia is fixed by the grounded foot, only the upper tibia moves, resulting in knee extension.

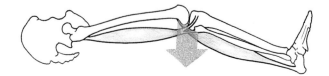

In Stomach Massage, the feet are fixed by the bar; the hamstrings therefore act to extend the knee. They work most often in synergy with the gastrocnemius, a knee flexor.*

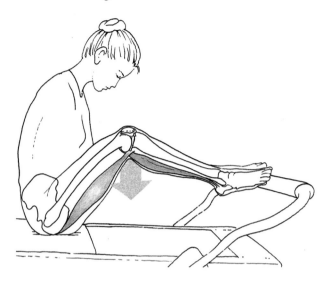

This effect is even more pronounced because the extension of the knee is made against the resistance of the springs. In the course of this exercise, the hamstrings initiate some movements and are themselves stretched by other movements.

What Happens to the Hamstrings in Stomach Massage?

Simultaneous contraction and stretching of the hamstrings during Stomach Massage pulls the pelvis in two directions.

In a seated position with the legs straight, it is difficult or impossible for the majority of people to create or maintain the slight natural curve of the lumbar spine. It should be noted here that the lower back shouldn't be "taken hostage" by the hamstrings.

✦ Placing the feet on the bar (therefore a bit higher) augments hip flexion. This puts the hamstrings under more tension, which then tends to cause the pelvis to tip backward (retroversion).

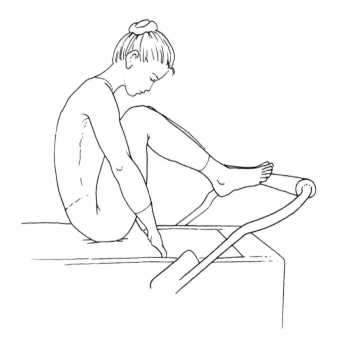

---

*For a more detailed analysis of knee flexion, see *Anatomy of Movement*, by Blandine Calais-Germain (Seattle: Eastland Press, 2007).

✦ Extending the legs then augments the hamstring stretch and the pelvis is pulled into more retroversion. Avoiding this requires intense recruitment of the back muscles.*

✦ Finally, when the feet are flexed, the stretch of the hamstrings is at its maximum. This is a critical moment in the exercise: we feel the calf muscle (the gastrocnemius) stretch. And this also pulls on the hamstrings. Here, if the hamstrings are short, the pelvis is pulled into more retroversion.

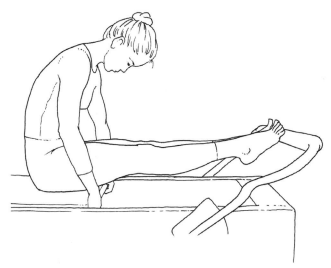

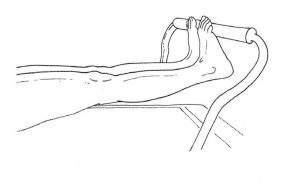

*We saw in chapter 1 that the back muscles, for the most part, antevert the pelvis and oppose the abdominals (primarily the rectus abdominus), which retrovert the pelvis.

Consequences

The Impact on the Lumbar Spine

The retroversion of the pelvis—caused by the pull of the hamstrings—in turn promotes flexion of the lumbar spine. This flexion isn't harmful in and of itself, but it takes place under pressure.

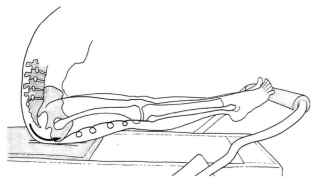

Where does the pressure come from? Pressure on the lumbar spine is partially caused by the load: the lumbar vertebrae are supporting the weight of the upper trunk. This is a very loaded position when the trunk and head are flexed over the legs.

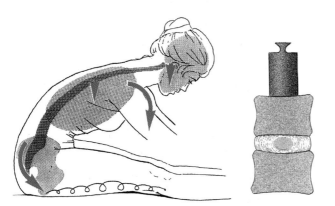

Pressure also occurs, in part, when the pelvic retroversion is caused by permanently tight hamstrings. And this occurs in a very specific context: the hamstrings are stretched, but they also contract, and this happens at the same time that we are moving the carriage in and out against spring resistance.

So, during flexion, the vertebrae are caught between two opposing forces and this can cause disk compression.

Disk Compression

Spinal flexion compresses the disks. We look specifically at what this action does to a disk's nucleus.

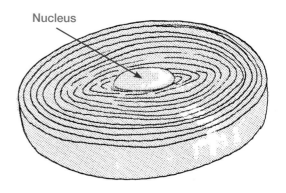

Nucleus

Flexion Pushes the Nucleus toward the Back

While yo-yoing of the pelvis causes "scissoring" of the annulus, prolonged compression of a lumbar disk when the spine is in flexion pushes the nucleus posteriorly.

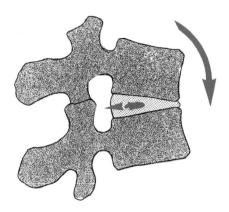

Vertebral Ligament and Sciatic Nerve

Pushing the nucleus posteriorly is much riskier than pushing it anteriorly, especially if the disk is already fragile, because in this area of the spinal column we find a ligament and components of the nervous system—in particular the sciatic nerve.

✦ If the nucleus has already broken through the annulus (and this rupture is usually posterior), this is called a *herniated disk*.

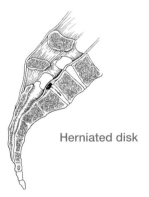

Herniated disk

✦ If the compression of the disk or the annulus puts pressure on the posterior ligaments, they can become overtaxed and painful. This can be a dull or a sharp pain, sometimes called *lumbago*.

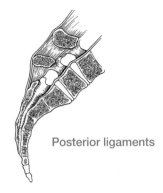

Posterior ligaments

✦ This compression can also irritate the sciatic nerve, creating the condition referred to as *sciatica*.

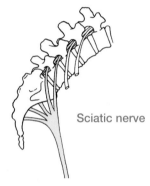

Sciatic nerve

All of these conditions—herniated disk, lumbago, and sciatica—can exist simultaneously.

When the disk is pinched posteriorly and stretched anteriorly (as it is in extension), the nucleus is pushed toward the front and toward the abdominal viscera. This is not undesirable and does not generally lead to disk herniations or sciatica. On the other hand, when the disk is squeezed in the front and open in the back (as it is in flexion), the nucleus is pushed posteriorly again, with all of the consequences that have been noted above.

Solutions and Prevention

How to Maintain the Integrity of the Vertebral Disks

There are a number of simple steps that can be taken to protect the vertebral disks during a Pilates routine.

1. Evaluate and Relax the Hamstrings

The best way to prepare for the Stomach Massage exercise is to learn just how tight the hamstrings are. To do this, sit on the floor with your legs straight in front of you. If you can maintain the lumbar curve even with your knees extended (1), you can probably perform this exercise without difficulty. However, in most cases, the hamstrings are too short and tight and the lumbar spine rounds (2). If this is the case, it's best to "prepare" the hamstrings with an exercise independent of, and prior to, Stomach Massage.

It's beneficial to lie on your back when stretching the hamstrings. Keep one foot on the floor, knee bent, and lift the other leg. Place a band around the raised foot, bending the knee if necessary. Try to bring your coccyx to the floor and your heel toward the ceiling as you gradually extend the knee (3).

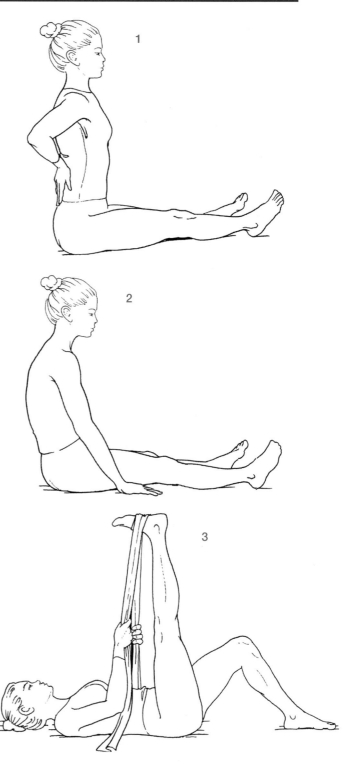

2. Stretch the Hamstrings on the Reformer

Lie down on the carriage with your feet in the straps. Straighten your legs out at a 45° angle from the table, with the heels connected and legs slightly turned out. Bring the legs to vertical while keeping the pelvis stable and the ischia parallel to the carriage.

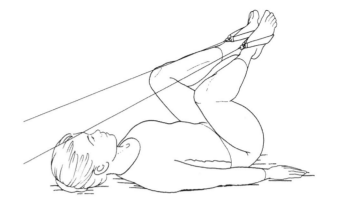

When the hamstrings are tight, this variation of Frog allows you to stretch to your threshold and then gradually move beyond it as you progressively work to bring the legs to vertical. Don't focus on reaching the 90° angle, but work to find a better range of motion. You can also use the roller and small balls to stretch the muscles and fascia.

3. Modify the Exercise

Before doing the Round Back variation of Stomach Massage, you can choose one of the variations in which the back is kept in alignment. In these variations, the arms and hands are placed behind you, allowing you to find the support you need to keep the spine straight. Once this step is mastered, you can progress to the full exercise. You can also place a ball between the shoulder blades and the lower back to support the lumbar spine.

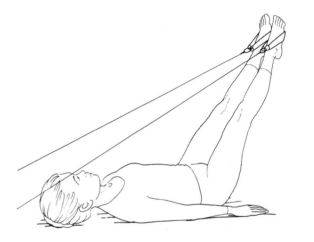

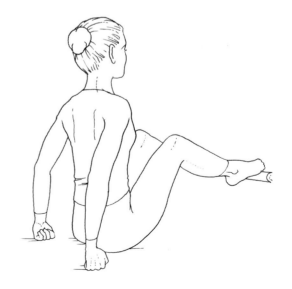

4. Open the Ribs

As in Teaser (see chapter 2), opening the ribs lessens the descent of the visceral mass and "lifts" the trunk. However, this doesn't lessen the pressure on the disks very much.

5. Reduce the Number or the Strength of the Springs

We can reduce the force of the springs, but remember that there needs to be at least minimal resistance, or the exercise will be too difficult to execute. Another option is to lower the bar, or simply to eliminate the exercise if it is too problematic.

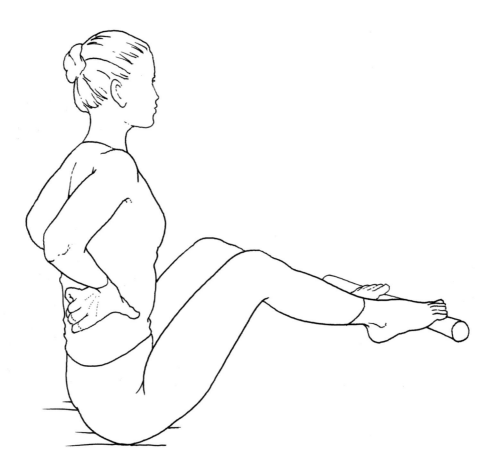

Other Exercises That Carry Similar Risks for the Lumbar Disks

Reformer Exercises

In principle, all of the Roll-up-type exercises load the spine and are capable of creating disk fatigue. So while the yo-yo effect "scissors" the annulus, exercises such as Stomach Massage cause instead an undesirable effect on the nucleus. Therefore it's not surprising to see exercises in this category that call for spinal flexion, like the Teaser. All the pressure directed toward the perineum also falls on the nucleus.

Short Box, Tree

Lifting the leg to a vertical position while seated behind the ischia will immediately cause flexion of the lumbar spine.

Tendon Stretch

The "V" position immediately pushes the disks to the back of the vertebral bodies.

Rowing Series: From the Hip

Here, as in the Crunch, flexion of the lumbar spine pushes the nucleus to the back.

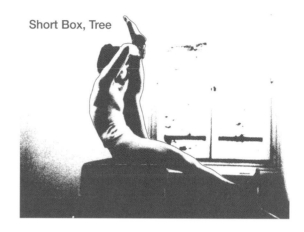

Short Box, Tree

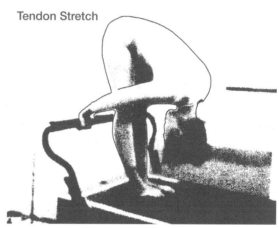

Tendon Stretch

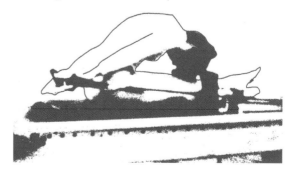

Rowing Series: From the Hip

Stork

If it is not done carefully, the act of bringing the thigh toward the chest can unnecessarily exaggerate flexion in the last lumbar vertebra.

Stork

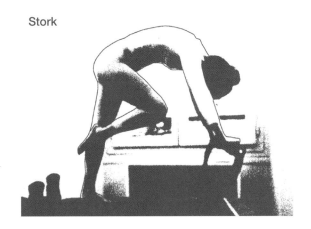

Mat Exercises

Mat exercises that require flexion of the spine from the head will have the same effect as similar exercises on the Reformer. The factors that cause the nucleus to move posteriorly in the vertebral bodies are the same as those that cause pressure on the perineum. We can therefore revisit all of the exercises that we covered in chapter 2, from the standpoint of how they reverse the lumbar curve and affect the spinal disks.

Roll-up (Spine Stretch Forward)

Here, the "hinge" effect forces the flexion into the lowest lumbar area, which isn't mobile in this type of movement.

Neck Pull

This version of the Roll-up emphasizes bringing the trunk farther forward over the legs. This position offsets the center of gravity even more and increases both the pressure on the discs and the tendency to push the nucleus posteriorly.

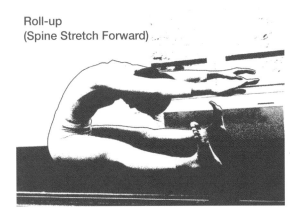

Roll-up
(Spine Stretch Forward)

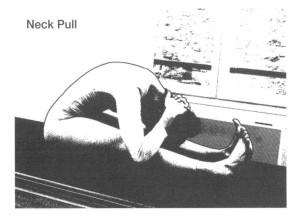

Neck Pull

Seal (Rolling Like a Ball)

The form of this rolling exercise—with the legs lifted—resembles the starting position of Stomach Massage and creates the same effects. Note that the first phase of this exercise, when we roll toward the head, is not a problem for the spinal disks; rather, it is the return phase that can negatively impact the lumbar spine.

Open-Leg Rocker

In this exercise, the position of the pelvis behind the ischia is almost necessary to maintain balance, but it immediately causes flexion of the lumbar spine and intensifies the load on that area.

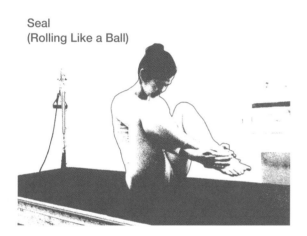

Seal
(Rolling Like a Ball)

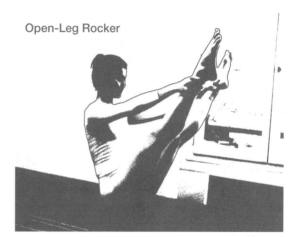

Open-Leg Rocker

4
ELEPHANT
and Pressure on the Wrist

This exercise, which is one of the basics of Pilates, generates repeated pressure on an area that is not able to support it.

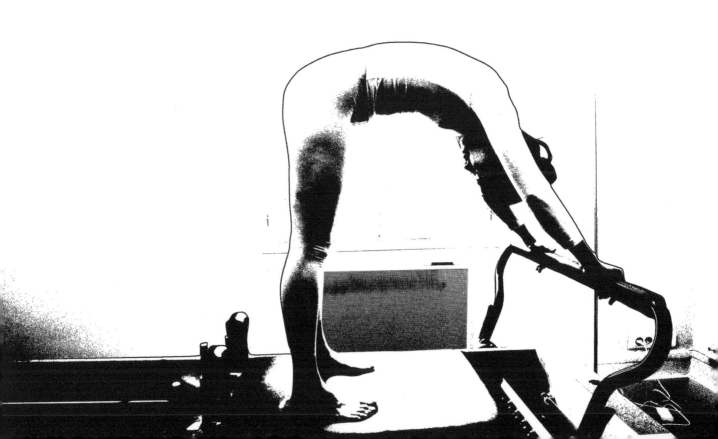

Principles of the Exercise

Starting Position

The feet are positioned on the carriage, either against the shoulder rests or more forward, depending on how flexible the ankles are. The hands are on the bar, supporting a lot of the body's weight. The head is positioned lower than the trunk, which is in flexion. The hips are also extremely flexed.

The Movement

In the outward movement, the feet move away from the hands—but not too much. The flexion of both the hips and the trunk is reduced. This movement is made against the resistance of the carriage and springs.

The return brings the feet closer to the hands again, and the flexion of the hips and trunk is increased. The amplitude of the movement is minimal because it is limited by the tightness of the hamstrings.

Observations

In this exercise, we put prolonged pressure on the front of the wrists. Sometimes this causes the bones of the wrist to feel stressed or creates a tingling feeling in the fingers. Why?

Because the many bones and tendons in the wrist are relatively exposed and vulnerable to damage.

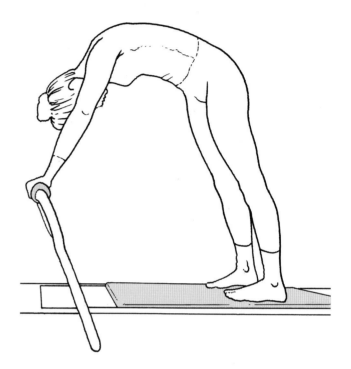

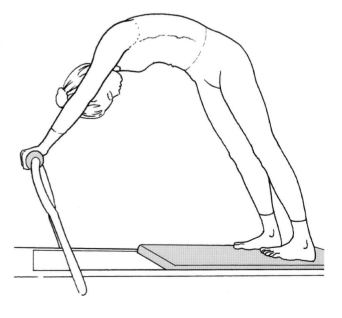

Anatomical Landmarks

The Wrist— a Joint with Many Bones

The wrist is not a joint that unites two bones (like, for example, the hip), but an articular region that joins fifteen very different bones:

+ the two bones of the forearm—the radius and ulna
+ the eight carpal bones, which are arranged in two rows
+ the five metacarpals

> The eight carpal bones lie in two rows. The first row is antebrachial and matches up with the forearm; the second row is metacarpal and matches up with the base of the metacarpals.

The Wrist Has Two Support Areas

When we put pressure on the wrists, there are two different places that are able to support the body's weight for short periods of time.

The First Support Area— Close to the Forearm

While doing the Elephant, we can put our weight on an area of support close to the forearm. To see this area on your own arm, bend the elbow and look at the palm side of your hand as you bend the hand slightly toward you (supinate). You will see several transverse folds in this area of the wrist.

The first support area is the zone about one centimeter beyond the crease closest to the hand. Here, we are on the second row of carpal bones, which consists of six bones aligned from the ulnar (little finger) side to the thenar (thumb) side. These six bones are the pisiform, triquetrum bone, hamate bone, capitate bone, trapezoid, and trapezium.

Like the first row of carpals, this second row of bones forms a kind of gutter that is hollowed at the front. Nine tendons (detailed on page 47) and the median nerve pass through this grooved area and are held together by a ligamentous band called the anterior annular ligament. This entire hollow, narrow area is called the *carpal tunnel*.

Generally, the carpal tunnel does not pro-

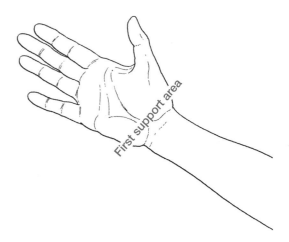

First support area

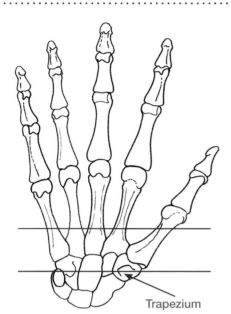

Trapezium

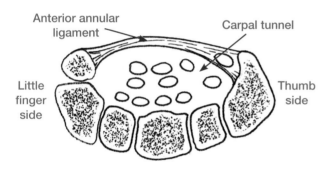

Anterior annular
ligament

Carpal tunnel

Little
finger
side

Thumb
side

Carpal tunnel viewed in cross section (depending
on the level of the cut, the groove is formed
by four, five, or six bones, but no matter the
number of bones, we will always find that the
area is grooved).

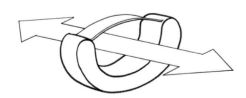

vide very good support for the body's weight.
This area is delicate because it's made up of
many small bones and other varied components. Furthermore, the skin in this area of
the body is thin, unlike other areas that are
designed for more pressure, like the heels or
the ischia, where the skin and underlying layers are thicker.

The Second Support Area—
the Border of the Palm

While doing the Elephant exercise, we can
support ourselves on a second area of the wrist
that lies close to the palm.

When we bend the elbow and look at
the hand in supination, we find this area just
beyond the first support area, right where the
palm starts. Here, the hand is a bit broader and
fleshier. This is where the bodies of the metacarpals start. The tendons are less grouped
here and have begun to separate toward their
respective fingers. Here also are the branched
endings of the median nerve, which serve the
hand. The anterior annular ligament doesn't
extend into this area; rather, there is a fibrous
web called the *medial palmar aponeurosis*.

The muscle mass at the base of the palm is a group of small muscles, called *intrinsic* because they originate and terminate in the hand itself.

By contrast, the tendons that pass through the carpal tunnel in this area are called *extrinsic* because they belong to muscles that lie outside of the hand in the forearm.

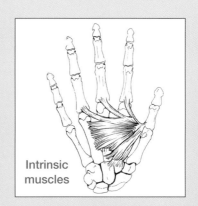

Intrinsic muscles

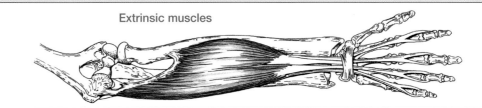

Extrinsic muscles

This second area is a more suitable support for the weight of the body than the carpal bones discussed above, because the greater muscle mass of the palm lessens the impact of pressure on the structures below.

However, neither area is able to support the body's weight for very long without creating problems.

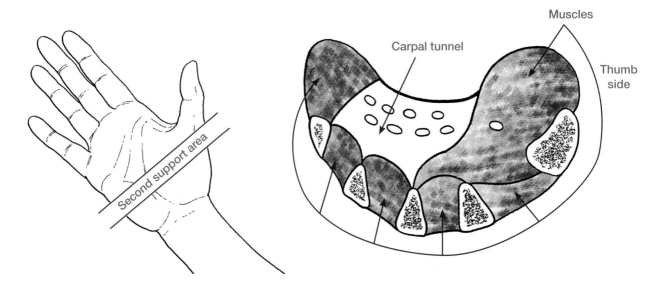

Second support area

Carpal tunnel

Muscles

Thumb side

Consequences

Positioning the Pressure

In each of the two support zones of the wrist that we've discussed, we can shift the pressure to the inside, middle, or outside. In each position, we find anatomical elements that make the additional pressure more or less acceptable.

The Carpal Area: The Three Regions of the First Zone

The inside (little finger side), middle, and outside (thumb side) regions of the carpal zone each have their strengths and weaknesses.

Pressure on the Little Finger Side

On the inside (little finger side) of the wrist, we find the process of the hamate bone and/or the pisiform bone (depending on whether we are closer to the palm or the wrist), both of which can be sensitive.

The hamate and pisiform bones can cause problems for three reasons:

+ These bones are almost directly under the skin.
+ The annular ligament and two intrinsic muscles of the little finger are attached to them.
+ The cubital nerve (which innervates the little finger) terminates on the external edge of this area. Repeated pressure on it can cause tingling in the little finger.

Pressure in the Middle

In the middle of the carpal tunnel, we find the tendons of four fingers bound in tight, superimposed layers. They are enveloped in a common sheath that is filled with a lubricating fluid.

Prolonged pressure on this area can cause compression of the tendons and of the fluid, which then can't circulate properly within the sheath.

The median nerve runs through the most external area of this middle area. Its compression can result in tingling or pain in the palm and the last four fingers.

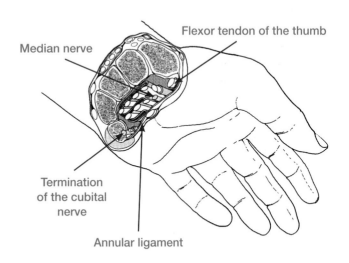

Median nerve

Flexor tendon of the thumb

Termination of the cubital nerve

Annular ligament

Details of the first zone of pressure

Pressure on the Thumb Side

Here, we put pressure on the trapezium bone, which may not be desirable for four reasons:

+ The bone is almost directly under the skin.
+ The annular ligament is attached to it, as well as the intrinsic muscles of the thumb.
+ The flexor tendon of the thumb—in its own sheath that contains a lubricating fluid—passes behind the annular ligament.
+ The median nerve is found in the innermost part of this area; repeated pressure can compress the nerve and cause tingling in the palm and the first four fingers.

The Base of the Palm: The Three Regions of the Second Zone

In general, the areas of this second zone are somewhat stronger than those of the first zone and are better able to withstand the body's pressure.

Pressure on the Little Finger Side

In this area, the bone is not directly under the skin, so pressure falls instead on the three small muscles that lead to the little finger.

Although pressure is better tolerated here than it is in the first zone, over time it can irritate the cubital nerve, which terminates between these muscles. Such irritation can cause tingling and numbness in certain fingers.

Pressure in the Middle

The middle of the second zone lies at the base of the third metacarpal, extending a bit on either side beneath the second and fourth metacarpals as well. In this area, the median nerve divides and leads to the fingers. The tendons are still in two superimposed layers, but they are not as tight, and the common sheath—filled with a lubricating fluid—is less restrictive.

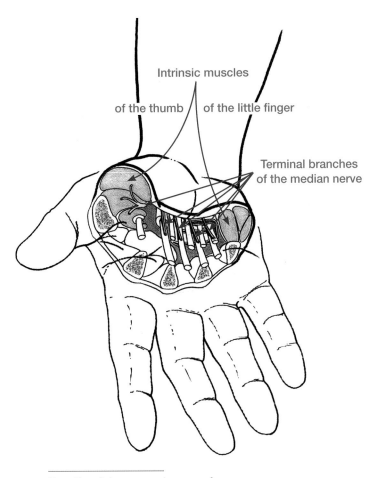

Intrinsic muscles

of the thumb / of the little finger

Terminal branches
of the median nerve

Details of the second zone of pressure

Prolonged pressure on this area can cause compression of the tendons and restriction of the lubricating fluid so that it doesn't circulate as well in the sheath. Repeated pressure can also cause tingling and numbness of the muscles of the fingers. However, the area is more protected because of the thick fascia in this region, which surrounds the muscles of the little finger and the thumb.

Pressure on the Thumb Side

In this area, the pressure falls on the mass of muscles at the base of the thumb, which provides a level of protection. The terminal branches of the median nerve pass between these muscles, and here too, repeated pressure can cause tingling and numbness, even though the pressure is cushioned by muscle tissue.

Solutions and Prevention

Shift the Body Weight Around

Because none of the support areas of the wrists are able to withstand pressure for very long, the key to preventing wrist problems is to continually shift the body weight around: from zone to zone, area to area, wrists to feet, etc.

1. Alternate Pressure between Zones One and Two

We have seen in the previous pages that the second zone is better able to withstand pressure than the first zone. Nevertheless, neither area can really support prolonged pressure. One solution is to constantly alternate pressure between the two zones.

The ability to switch between the two areas depends on the angle formed by the forearms and the bar that the hands are supported on. This angle is going to change depending on:

+ the height of the bar, which is adjustable on many Reformers;
+ whether the weight of the trunk is more over the feet or more forward over the hands; and
+ the flexibility of the hamstrings.

It is therefore helpful to vary the position of the body in relationship to the equipment, even slightly, to change the point of pressure.

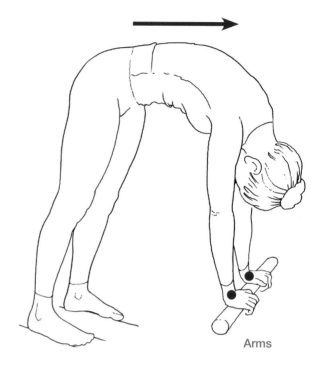

Arms

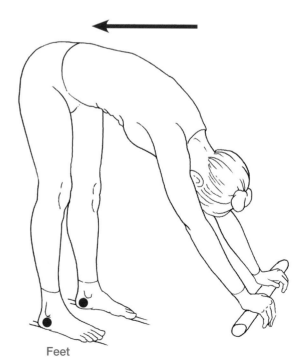

Feet

2. Switch Pressure among the Inner, Middle, and Outer Sections of Each Zone

Here, shifting the pressure depends on the angle formed between the forearms and the hands—not in the sagittal plane, but in the frontal plane.

We can modify this angle by separating the hands more or by bringing them closer together on the bar: when the hands are placed farther apart, the pressure is more to the inside, while placing the hands closer together brings the pressure toward the outside.

Note that it's not necessary to move the hands very much to change the pressure, and that we can make these small changes constantly. We can even position the hands asymmetrically depending on what we feel in the wrists; it's not necessary to maintain a symmetrical position to perform this exercise.

3. Alternate between Pressure and No Pressure

Between repetitions, or whenever possible, we can place the weight of the trunk more over the feet and let the tissues of the wrist take a break.

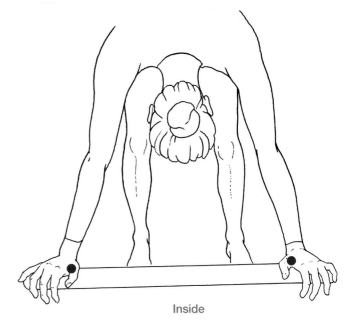

Inside

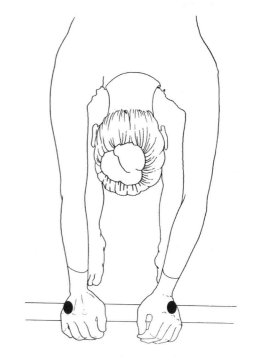

Outside

Actively Orient the Forearms to Find the Best Place to Put Pressure

The choice of where we place the wrist or the hand can be determined by actively orienting the wrist. The muscles have tendons that extend to the hand and act like "reins" that can be synchronized. The wrist is braced and held by its musculature.

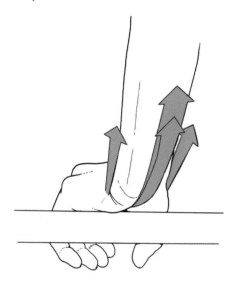

Strengthen the Elbow, Wrist, and Hand Simultaneously

This exercise strengthens the muscles of the forearms—including those around the elbow and the wrist—and the hands.*

With the fingers straight, place the fingertips of one hand on the fingertips of the other hand and press forcefully. To intensify the work, get down on your knees and place your fingertips on the floor, pressing them into the ground. If this isn't enough, put the pressure on the hands and feet and lift the knees off the floor.

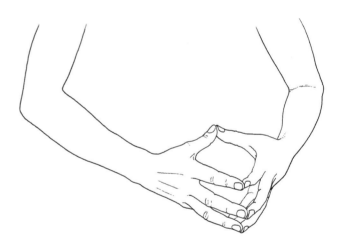

*For more information on ways to strengthen these muscles, see Blandine Calais-Germain's *Anatomy of Movement*.

Release the Muscles of the Entire Arm

This exercise stretches all of the tissues and muscles of the arm from the sternum to the ends of the fingers.* It is a continuation of the stretch initiated in the Elephant and is contra-indicated for those with shoulder problems.

Sitting on a stool, stretch one arm out behind you, extend the elbow and the wrist, open the palm, and separate all the fingers as wide as possible while placing them in extension.

Do the same thing with the other arm, then try it with both arms at the same time.

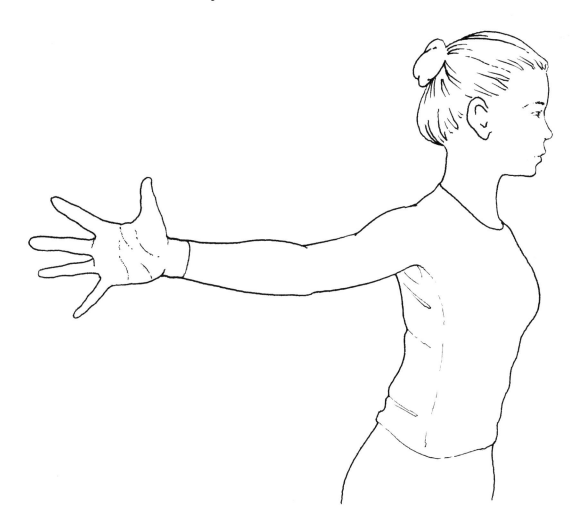

---

*For more information on releasing the muscles of the arms, see Blandine Calais-Germain's *Anatomy of Movement*.

Other Exercises That Present Similar Challenges to the Wrists

Reformer Exercises

When using the Reformer, it is helpful to remember that all the exercises done with the hands in the straps make it possible to choose the point of pressure, because the weight of the body is not on the hands.

In addition, there are many other Reformer exercises where the weight of the body is shared by the wrists and the lower limbs, allowing the user to control the pressure on the wrists.

Exercises Done with the Straps: Hundred, Coordination, Backstroke, Rowing Series, Teaser, Kneeling Arms, Chest Expansion

As in all of the exercises done with the straps (where the pressure is not as great as with Elephant), we have the luxury of finding a good position for each movement, usually in the second pressure zone. This is an opportunity to explore different ways of holding the handles or loops and to modify the shape of the hand, depending on what feels best.

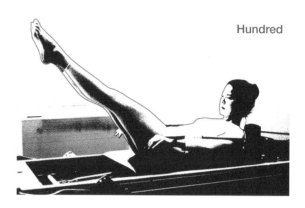

Hundred

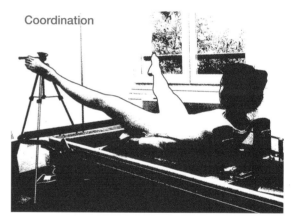

Coordination

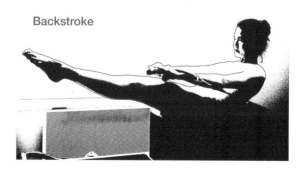

Backstroke

Rowing Series

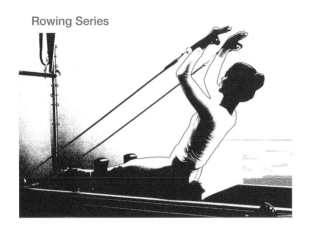

Kneeling Arms

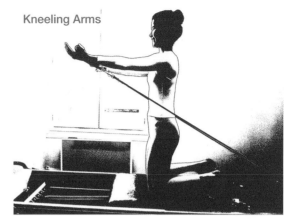

Chest Expansion

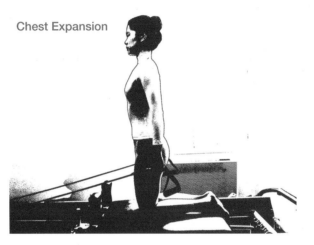

Exercises Using the Bar: Swan Prep, Stork

Swan Prep

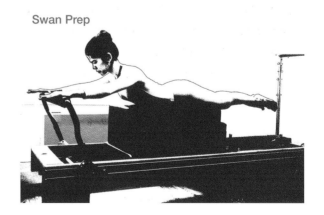

Lie prone on the box with your hands flat on the bar. Given that there is much less pressure on the hands when you go into spinal extension, you are at leisure to explore a variety of positions and to adjust your hands according to what you find. In Stork, which is a variation of Elephant with one leg lifted, you have the same position options that we've offered for Elephant.

Mat Exercises

Compared to the Reformer, mat work has fewer exercises that require supporting yourself on your hands. All of them are done with the hands in extension.

Leg Pull Back

Leg Pull Back (also called Leg Pull-up) is a variation of Leg Pull Front (also called Leg Pull-down) done with the back toward the floor. This exercise puts a huge demand on the wrists and requires good shoulder-girdle stability. In fact, because of the position, more of the body weight is supported by the hands than the feet.

Kneeling Side Kick

This whole series is done with the weight on one hand and one knee. It calls for the same degree of control as Leg Pull Back, with the added challenge of maintaining balance.

Leg Pull Front

This is a version of Push-up done with the weight on the hands and the feet. It calls for a high degree of shoulder-girdle stability in order to minimize the pressure on the wrists.

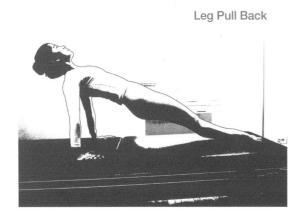

Leg Pull Back

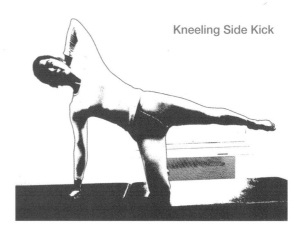

Kneeling Side Kick

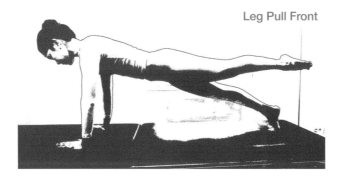

Leg Pull Front

5

LONG STRETCH

and Hyperextension of the Wrist

The Long Stretch series has several variations, all of which call for extension of the wrist.

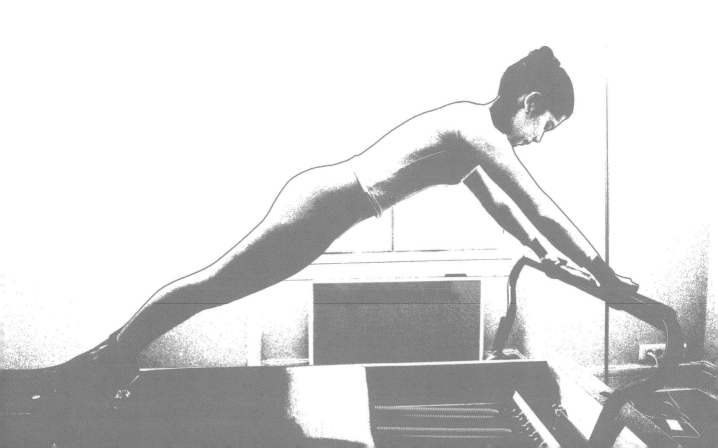

Principles of the Exercise

Starting Position

We start with the body in a plank position, with the hands on the bar and the fingers wrapped around it. The toes are placed at the center of the carriage in the groove of the headrest.

The trunk is not parallel to the carriage, but at an oblique angle: the shoulders are higher than the pelvis because the bar on which the hands are placed is higher than the carriage that supports the feet.

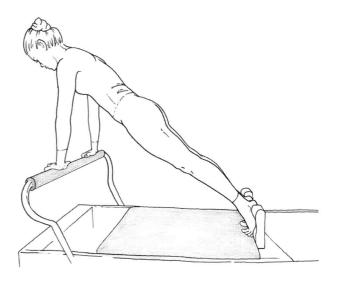

The Movement

The exercise consists of moving the carriage in and out while keeping the body aligned between the head and the heels. The pelvis needs to remain stable (without tilting in one direction or the other) on both the push-out and the return.

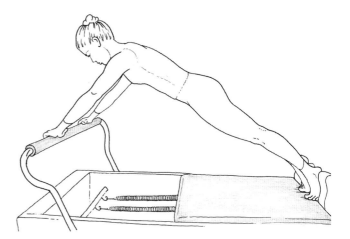

Observations

When we first perform the Long Stretch, it is very common to hyperextend the wrist, dropping it below the top of the Reformer bar. Why?

The stress is more on the wrist than on the ankle joint, especially at the beginning of the exercise. When we try to move the carriage, the angle of the wrist relative to the forearm changes and the wrist is put into forced extension. The farther the carriage goes from the starting position, the less pressure there is on the wrist. It is therefore at the start of the movement and at the end of the return when the wrist is under the most stress.

Anatomical Landmarks

The Wrist— a Naturally Weak Joint

As we discussed in the previous chapter, several features of the wrist combine to make it relatively weak, as well as vulnerable to injury.

Absence of Muscle Mass

The wrist lacks strength because no muscles cross the joint. Instead, it is crossed by tendons that originate in the forearm and extend to the hand and fingers.

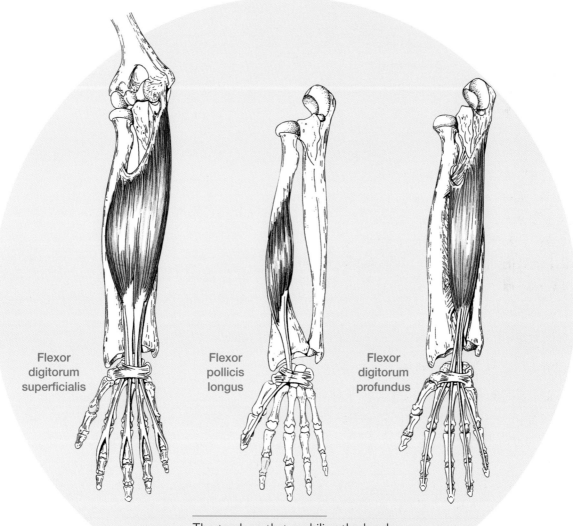

Flexor digitorum superficialis

Flexor pollicis longus

Flexor digitorum profundus

The tendons that mobilize the hand and wrist originate on muscles of the forearm and cross the wrist

An Area Very Dense with Tendons

The tendons that mobilize the hand and wrist originate on muscles of the forearm and cross the wrist. The tendons that pass in the front of the joint flex the wrist, while those that cross the back of it are used for extension. Tendons on either side of the wrist are used in lateral inclination. Each of these tendons can easily become irritated and painful.

The Joint Is Commonly Placed in Extension

The wrist joint must frequently be stabilized to allow for optimal positioning of the fingers for action. The action position of the fingers is flexion, and the position of the wrist that best facilitates this position is slight extension (about 30°). This extension lightly stretches the tendons of the flexors, which, when put under tension, start to flex the fingers.

We also spontaneously extend the wrist and incline it a bit internally whenever we grab something, or prepare to grab something. We call this the *functional grip position*. When we look at the hand in this position from the back, we can see a slight transversal bend. In profile, we see that the forearm does not continue in a straight line from the back of the hand; rather, it forms about a 45° angle.

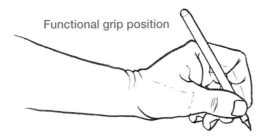
Functional grip position

The angle of wrist extension is the angle formed by the intersection of two lines: the first line follows the angle of the ulna, while the second line runs toward the ulna from the fifth metacarpal. The angle is measured where the two lines cross.

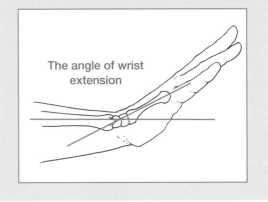
The angle of wrist extension

The Wrist in Hyperextension

The tendency of the wrist to go into extension predisposes its movement into another more extreme position, hyperextension. How do we recognize hyperextension? The angle increases to 60° and sometimes reaches 80°. The folds at the back of the joint are much more exaggerated.

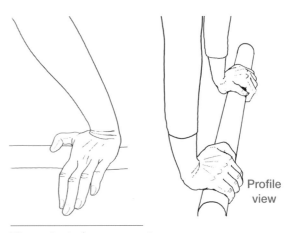
Profile view

The wrist in hyperextension

Consequences

Bone Compression

When the wrist is extended, the posterior areas of the bones of the first row of carpals come closer together in the back. In the front, the opposite occurs: the anterior parts separate.

In hyperextension, this effect is at its greatest. The posterior regions of the bones in the two rows compress. In the Long Stretch, the effect is even more dramatic because the bones are under extreme pressure, supporting almost half of the body's weight. This can create pain in the joint.

Stretching of the Anterior Components of the Wrist

When the wrist is hyperextended, all of the elements at the front of the joint are put under passive tension, including

+ the tendon of the flexor pollicis longus
+ the four tendons of the flexor digitorum profundus
+ the four tendons of the flexor digitorum superficialis
+ the sheath that wraps the tendons
+ the lubricating fluid within the sheath
+ the median nerve

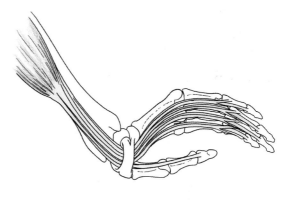

The tendons of the extrinsic muscles (represented here without the tendon sheath)

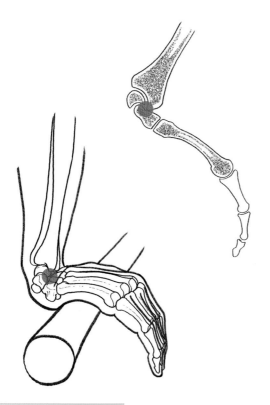

Bone compression at the wrist

The median nerve is one of three nerves of the hand. It arises from the spinal cord at the cervical vertebrae and emerges from the hollow of the armpit. From there, it travels the length of the upper arm, then down the middle of the anterior forearm to arrive at the middle of the wrist, hence its name. From there, it branches to the front of the hand. It is both a motor and a sensory nerve, causing the muscle contractions that produce extension of the elbow, wrist, and fingers, as well as relaying sensory information.

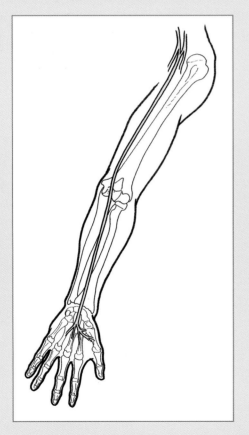

Repeated compression and stretching of the wrist over a period of time can cause tingling, itching, or a burning sensation in the hand.

Weakness of the Wrist and Shoulder-Girdle Instability

When we begin to practice the Long Stretch, a lack of strength in the wrist often becomes apparent—and often accompanies a general lack of muscle engagement in the entire upper limb.

Why? Because Long Stretch already requires intense recruitment of the trunk and leg muscles, while at the same time putting tremendous pressure on the hands. In principle, the trunk should remain absolutely stable; the only movement should come from the shoulder girdle, which acts to brake the movement and also to bring the weight of the trunk back to the home position.

A beginner usually has a hard time just maintaining control, however, and this almost always means that placement of the upper extremities will suffer. Because the placement of the hands on the bar is not a matter of choice, they tend to push or pull other parts of the body into specific positions:

+ The wrist "falls" on the bar in passive extension.
+ At the same time, the elbows lock into passive extension, or passive hyperextension.
+ The shoulder girdle receives the counterforce from the bar, transmitted from the hand to the entire upper extremity. This counterforce can cause the shoulder blades to move in three ways: the shoulder blades move toward the ears, the shoulder blades move toward each other, and the shoulder blades "wing" and the medial edges move toward the ceiling.

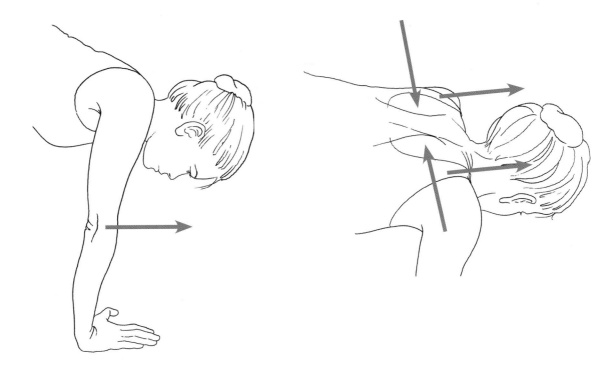

Solutions and Prevention

How to Avoid Hyperextension of the Wrist

With a little bit of care, we can protect the wrists and avoid hyperextension during the Long Stretch and other similar exercises.

1. Find the Best Angle for the Wrist

We need to recognize the most functional extension position of the wrist when it is not under pressure.

To find this angle, first align the hand with the forearm (1). We see that the fingers open a bit (which means the joints are slightly in extension). Starting from this position, we can see how the wrist goes into extension as we progressively bend the third (middle), fourth (ring), and fifth (little) fingers until they are one centimeter from the palm, or touching it (2).

The angle of the wrist is not the same for everyone. Once we find this optimal angle, we can try to duplicate it even when the wrist is under pressure on the bar.

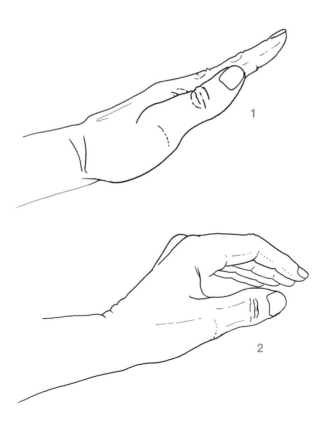

2. Reinforce the Wrist Joint

We can strengthen the muscles of the wrist joint by giving resistance successively to its four surfaces.

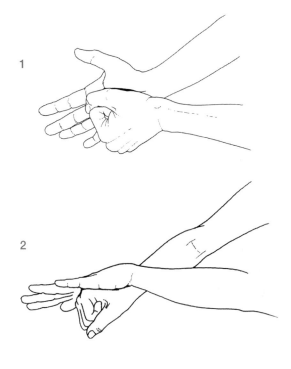

+ Place the fist of one hand against the palm of the other (1), and resist the mutual pressure equally with both hands. For the hand in a fist (this is the one where we observe the work), this is working the flexors of the wrist. If we do the opposite and press the open hand against the back of the fist (2), we see the wrist extensors working.

+ Next place the thumb or little finger side of the closed fist against the palm of the opposite hand (3 and 4). This reinforces the lateral muscles of the forearm and their tendons that cross the wrist.

+ Repeat this sequence several times until the wrist feels steady. Then change the role of the hands.*

+ If we want to work more intensely, we can do what we did when preparing for the Elephant. Kneeling on the floor, put pressure on the hands while keeping the fingers straight. This strengthens the muscles of the hands and the forearms.

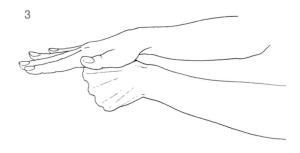

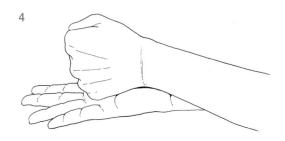

---

*For more details of this exercise, see Blandine Calais-Germain's *Anatomy of Movement*.

3. Stabilize the Shoulder Blades, Guide the Wrist from the Shoulder

Maintaining scapular stability during Long Stretch means keeping the shoulder blades from rising and collapsing toward each other. The principle muscles in play here are the serratus anterior, which keeps the shoulder blades on their respective sides of the thorax, and the pectoralis major, which lowers the clavicle. These two muscles work to fix the shoulder blades, which facilitates more accurate placement of the arms and elbows. Then, the elbow should be slightly "fixed" by the anterior flexors, which keep it from hyperextending. Finally, the wrist is able to retain the proper amount of extension, held in place by the same muscles that are overstretched if we let it go into hyperextension.

4. Redistribute the Body Weight

Since the weight of the body is more on the wrists than on the feet at the start of the exercise, it's helpful to redistribute this weight throughout the movement. For instance, you can try to push the carriage more with your feet to alleviate pressure on the upper extremities. On the return, try to oppose the force of the springs with your feet rather than with your arms and hands.

5. Relax the Wrists in Flexion

Between exercises, we can place the forearms over the bar for support and let the wrists go into passive flexion, which will relax the entire anterior surface.

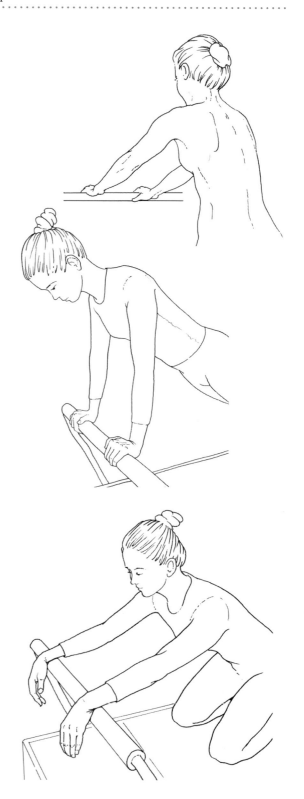

Other Exercises That Present Similar Challenges to the Wrists

Reformer Exercises

Hyperextension of the wrist is often a result of trying to find the force in an exercise, and it is especially common when an exercise calls for an extra boost of power from the upper extremities or when the arms are supporting the bulk of the weight. As in the preceding chapter, we can separate those exercises done with the straps from those that require direct pressure on the wrists.

Exercises Done with the Straps: Kneeling Arm Series (Shave the Head)

In this series done on the knees, one of the exercises calls for placing the hands (while in the straps or handles) behind, or close to, the head, and then lengthening the arms out. This movement requires a force that encourages extension of the wrist. If this happens, care should be taken to modify the movement or to break it down into simpler steps. The illustration shown here is one example of a simpler version of the exercise.

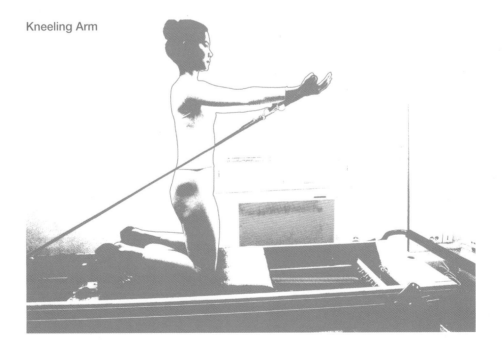

Kneeling Arm

*Exercises Done with Direct Pressure
on the Wrists: Knees Off,
Tendon Stretch*

In Knees Off (one of the Knee Stretch series), the majority of the body's weight is on the wrists. Opening and closing of the carriage is done with the feet on the carriage and the knees raised. The pressure on the upper extremities often causes the wrists to hyper-extend, the shoulder blades to rise, and the elbows to lock in hyperextension. The same effects are noted in Tendon Stretch because there, too, the weight is supported by the upper extremities. We look to ameliorate this effect by stabilizing the shoulder blades, strengthening the wrists, and exploring the different ways of adjusting the pressure.

Knees Off

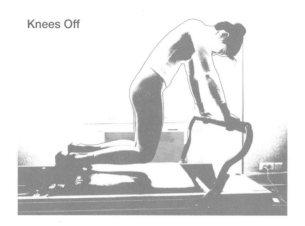

Tendon Stretch

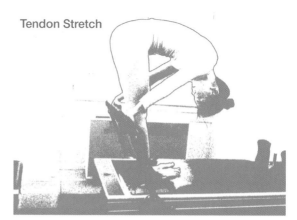

Mat Exercises

In the mat work, there are fewer exercises that put this kind of pressure on the wrists, but they all start with the hand in extension. In addition, the most advanced exercises (such as Shoulder Bridge and Bicycle) require that the hips be supported by the hands—which are in extension.

Leg Pull Front

This variation on Push-up, where the weight is on the hands and the feet, requires stability of the shoulder blades in order to lessen the pressure on the wrist joint.

Leg Pull Front

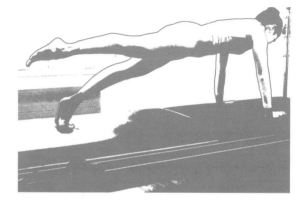

Kneeling Side Kick

This whole series is done with the weight on one hand and one knee. It calls for the same degree of control as Leg Pull Back, with the added challenge of maintaining balance.

Mermaid Stretch

This is a lateral flexion exercise with the knees on the mat and one hand on the floor at the side. The hand is in extension and under pres-sure, especially when we go up on the knees. As in the previous exercises, it is necessary to take the same precautions. You can also choose to make a fist with the supporting hand, or place the fingertips on the floor.

Leg Pull Back

A variation of Leg Pull Front, this exercise engages the wrist even more and requires excellent shoulder-girdle stability.

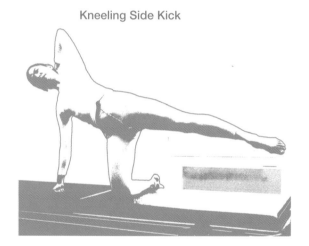

Kneeling Side Kick

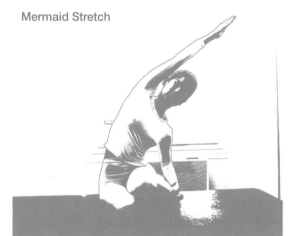

Mermaid Stretch

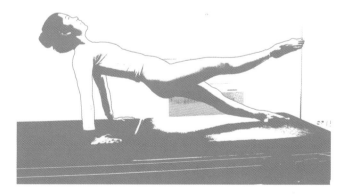

Leg Pull Back

6

DOWN STRETCH

and Lumbar Hyperextension

In this exercise, the lowest area of the spine tends to be pulled into extreme extension.

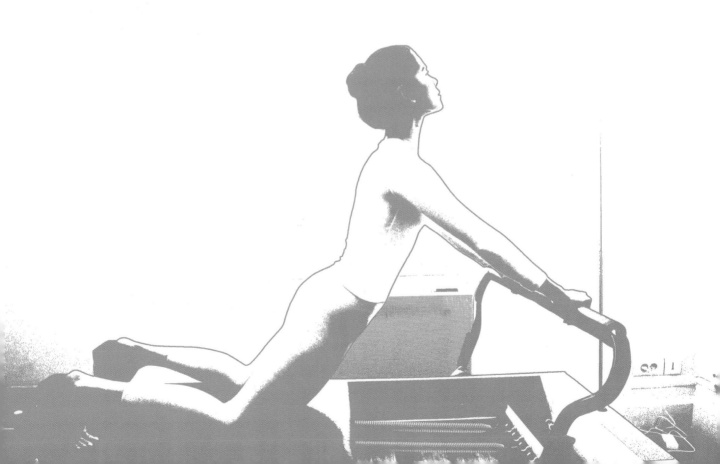

Principles of the Exercise

Starting Position

The knees are on the carriage, and the soles of the feet are against the shoulder rests, with heels reaching backward and toes turned toward the front of the Reformer. The pelvis is brought forward toward the hands, which are on the bar. The back is in thoracic and lumbar extension.

The Movement

Pressing the hands and feet against their respective supports, we try to push the carriage out and then control the return, while maintaining a constant and appropriate level of extension of the thoracic and lumbar spine. The back should stay in moderate extension while opening the carriage as well as on the return.

Observations

In the course of this exercise, the extension tends to increase past the level that is appropriate, especially in the lumbar spine. Why?

Because the joint between L5 and S1 is particularly vulnerable to several kinds of instability.

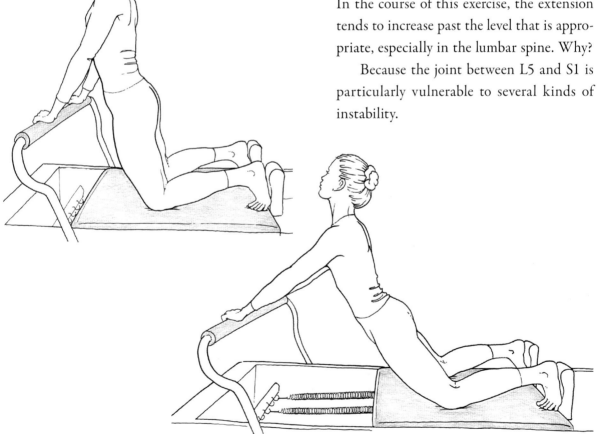

Anatomical Landmarks

L5/S1: A Junction That Is Particularly Mobile in Extension

The junction of L5 and S1 is predisposed to hyperextension for the following reasons:

+ The body of the fifth lumbar vertebra is lower in the back than in the front, therefore its surfaces are not parallel.
+ The L5/S1 disk has the same profile—thinner at the back than at the front.
+ The sacral plateau is inclined to the front at about 30° (this varies depending on the individual).
+ The slightly protruding spinous processes of L5 and the sacrum don't inhibit extension. (This is in contrast to the long and downward-slanted processes of the thoracic spine, which inhibit extension in the thoracic area when they meet.)

All of these factors combine to dispose the lumbosacral junction to extension, rather than flexion—more than in any other region of the lumbothoracic. When we perform an extension exercise like Down Stretch, this area tends to collapse, meaning that it over-arches or hyperextends.

This isn't to say that this arch should be avoided altogether, but it is important to note that in any exercise that forces the lumbar spine

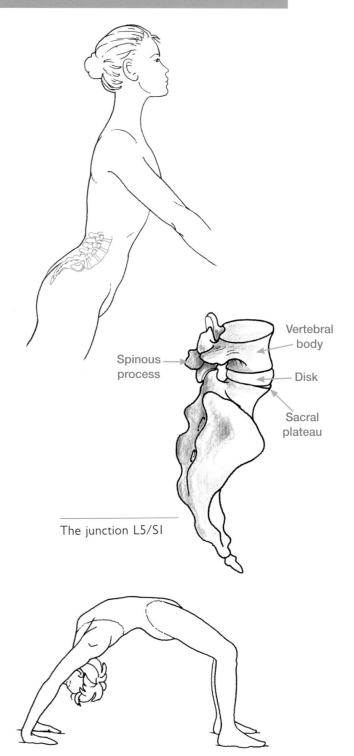

Vertebral body

Spinous process

Disk

Sacral plateau

The junction L5/S1

into extension, the maximum amplitude will be reached very easily—especially in beginners.

L5/S1 and the Upright Position

The lumbosacral junction supports a heavy load because it carries the weight of the upper body: the trunk, the head and neck, and the upper extremities.

When the weight arrives at the sacral plateau, it can be divided into two forces:

+ a pressure that is exerted **perpendicularly** on the plateau that helps keep the junction stable
+ another that is exerted **parallel** to the plateau, which tends to push the vertebral body of L5 forward and downward

L5 is held in place by the contact between its inferior articular processes and the facets of S1. (The figure at right shows only the articulation on the right side, but in reality there are two—symmetrical and situated at the back of the vertebra.) If the second (parallel) force is too strong, it can cause excessive pressure and irritation on the articular cartilage of the facets, which are very small. In turn, this irritation can cause a localized inflammation, which can itself put pressure on the nerves in the area (sciatic nerve, crural nerve). Although the cause is different, it can result in the same problems that we discussed in chapter 1.

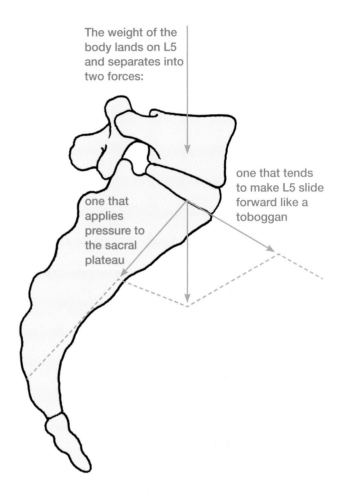

The weight of the body lands on L5 and separates into two forces:

one that tends to make L5 slide forward like a toboggan

one that applies pressure to the sacral plateau

The Lumbosacral Junction and Anteversion

Everything that contributes to the inclination of the sacral plateau intensifies the second force—in particular, anteversion of the pelvis and everything that causes anteversion.

Consequences

The Pelvis Is Predisposed to Anteversion

When the lower spine is unstable, the muscles and ligaments of the pelvis absorb more strain.

Stretching the Rectus Femoris Leads to Pelvic Anteversion

The rectus femoris is a thigh muscle that inserts on the iliac bone, crosses the hip joint, and descends to the knee, which it also crosses. This biarticular muscle moves two joints: it flexes the hip and extends the knee. It is one of the quadricep muscles, but the other three only flex the hip.

We explained in chapter 1 that stretching the hip flexors pulls the pelvis into anteversion. In Down Stretch it is the rectus femoris that causes this anteversion. The muscle is put under tension not only by the extension of the hip, but by the combination of knee flexion with hip extension:

✦ Hip extension (1) stretches the upper insertion.
✦ Knee flexion (2) stretches the lower insertion.

This stretching turns the two muscles into one, which pulls on the pelvis all the more because it tends to be tight and short. This pulls the pelvis into anteversion (3).

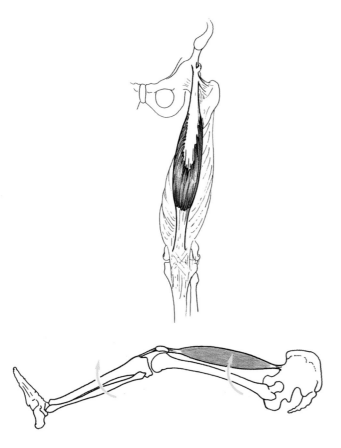

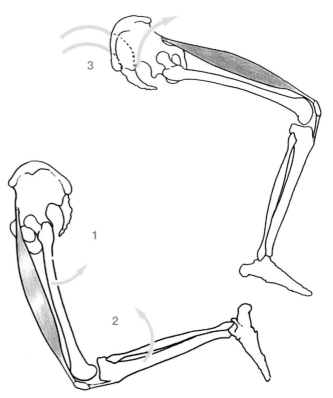

While the stretching we discussed in chapter 1 was passive, Down Stretch forces the rectus femoris to be very active: it works to retain knee flexion while the trunk and pelvis are tilting.

Shortened Hip Ligaments Can Tilt the Pelvis

A tight rectus femoris isn't the only factor that causes anteversion of the pelvis. Short hip ligaments are also responsible for the involuntary tilting of the pelvis.

The hip joint (composed of the iliac bone and the femur) is held together by a thick capsule that is reinforced by ligaments (especially the anterior ligaments). These ligaments tend to shorten and dramatically limit hip extension, leaving the joint in permanent flexion. In a standing position, this means that the pelvis is pulled into anteversion, which creates an unwanted lordosis of the lumbar spine.

Therefore, before trying to correct an overly arched lumbar area, try to determine if it is caused by a tightness of the rectus femoris or by the anterior hip ligaments.

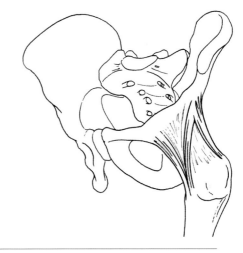

This capsule is reinforced by ligaments found especially at the front of the hip, where they are arranged in three bundles that together form an "N" shape.

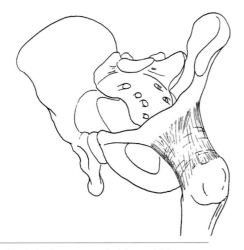

The hip joint is surrounded by a thick, strong capsule that is attached to the iliac bone and the femur.

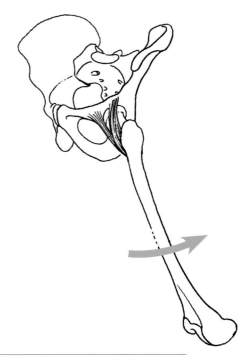

When the hip is extended, all of the anterior ligaments are put under tension.

How to Stabilize the Pelvis in Down Stretch

There are several ways to stabilize and protect the pelvis during Down Stretch and other similar exercises.

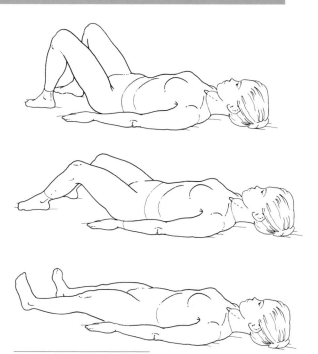

1. Identify the Point Where the Pelvis Tips Forward toward the Trunk

To identify this point, lie on your back on a mat. Your hips and knees should be flexed, and the pelvis should be in a neutral position (neither in anteversion nor in retroversion). Extend the legs on the mat and note exactly when the movement starts to pull the pelvis into anteversion.*

Identify the point

2. Oppose Pelvic Anteversion

Once we've found the point at which the pelvis tips, we can stabilize it in two ways:

Recruit the abdominal muscles: The principle abdominal muscle for this purpose is the rectus abdominus, because it's the muscle that brings the pelvis into retroversion. By finding the point at which anteversion starts to happen, we can measure out the right amount of contraction needed to control the pelvis throughout the exercise.

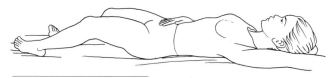

Recruit the abs

Use the gluteus maximus muscles: Anteversion of the pelvis can also be opposed by contracting the gluteus maximus muscles. These are the muscles that extend the hip if

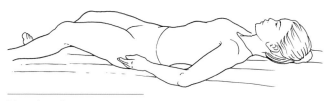

Use the glutes

the femur is free, and they are also powerful when used to retrovert the pelvis. They help create a sense of control that comes not just from the rectus abdominus and the front of the body but also from the back of the body.

---

*For more information on finding this point, see page 75 of Blandine Calais-Germain's *No-Risk Abs*.

3. Relax the Hips

In order to begin to relax the hips when the anterior ligaments are tight, we first should open the groin.

Lie down on your stomach (1), legs straight, and feel the crease of the hip under the hollow of the iliac bone (this hollow corresponds to the upper insertion of the rectus femoris). In the beginning, practice by trying to bring the iliac crests toward the floor. This retroversion can be done by contracting the glutes (shown here) or the rectus abdominus (not shown). Alternate making this movement with the glutes and then the abs. And then try it in a vertical position (2).

4. Stretch a Tight Rectus Femoris

Lie down on your stomach as in the previous exercise and take your right foot in your left hand. You will feel the hollow of the iliac bone change shape as the anteversion becomes more pronounced because of the strong knee flexion. From this position, try to bring the hip back to the floor by retroversing the pelvis with a gluteal or abdominal contraction. This action will put the rectus femoris under tension.

At this stage, you will feel a stretch at different levels of the muscle depending on where there is tightness. You can choose which areas to stretch:

+ If you focus on knee flexion, you will feel the stretch at the lower part of the muscle.
+ If you focus on retroversion, the stretch will be more predominant in the upper part of the muscle.

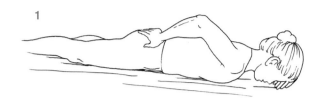

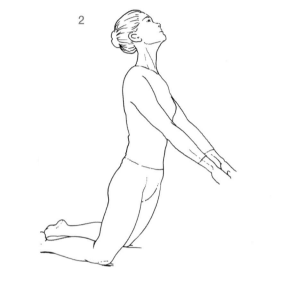

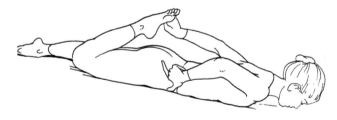

After you have stretched the muscles on the right side, change sides, so that you are holding your left foot in your right hand.

If the knee is fragile, place a band or strap around the front of the ankle to reduce the angle of flexion.

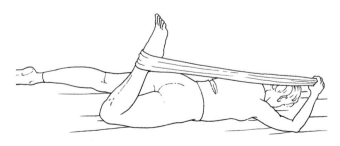

Other Exercises Where There Is a Risk of L5/S1 Hyperextension

Reformer Exercises

Down Stretch and the first two exercises listed below are basic exercises that risk hyperextending the lumbosacral joint. Snake is an advanced-level exercise that should not cause "involuntary" hyperextension because in principle the person performing the exercise should have already mastered stabilizing L5/S1. However, it is included here because such hyperextension is possible.

Swan Prep

Lie on the box on your belly, so that your body is parallel to the floor. Extend the whole body from the head to the feet. Here, the back goes into extension and it's at this moment that we risk reproducing the same situation that we find in Down Stretch.

Hamstring Curls

Lie facedown on the box with your arms crossed and the forehead resting on the arms. The straps are around the ankles and the knees are bent to about 45° to begin. The movement consists only of pulling the feet closer to the buttocks and then returning, but the effort is doubled here because the back is not supported by the pressure of the hands on

the bar. This is the same position we used to stretch the rectus femoris, and it makes the L5/S1 junction similarly vulnerable.

Swan Prep

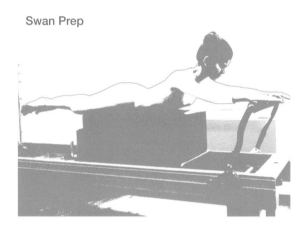

Hamstring Curls

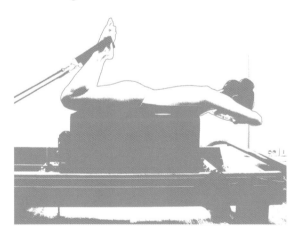

Snake

In this exercise, the hands are supported on one side of the carriage while the feet are at the other side of the Reformer. The head is aligned with the legs. As the arms push the carriage out, the trunk goes into extension between the two extremities. This creates a situation where the stress is focused on the L5/S1 junction.

Snake

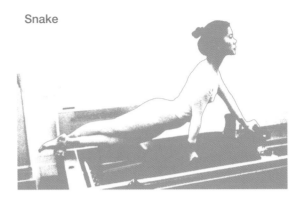

Knee Stretch (Arched)

In this exercise, the legs bend and open independently beneath the back, which is held in extension. It is especially when the legs are extended that we risk accentuating the extension at the L5/S1 hinge.

Knee Stretch (Arched)

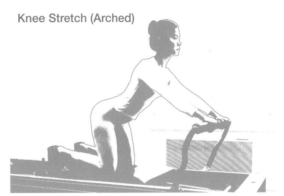

Mat Exercises

All of these exercises are done lying on the belly on the mat, except Shoulder Bridge, which is a version of the rectus femoris stretch that is done with the back on the mat.

Swimming

On the belly, the arms and legs make alternating scissor movements. To do this exercise correctly, the pelvis needs to be stable so that pressure isn't put on the lower back.

Swimming

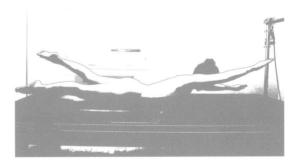

Single Leg Kick, Double Leg Kick

Like the previous exercise, this one starts on the belly, but we add knee flexion and extension. The exercise requires that you stabilize the pelvis and lower back without overtaxing the lumbar junction, which is likely to compensate for any weakness in the thoracic spine.

Shoulder Bridge

This version of the bridge stretches the rectus femoris. It is therefore imperative not to allow the L5/S1 junction to over-arch as you bring the pelvis up to the height of the knees.

Neck Roll

This variation of the Cobra forces the L5/S1 junction into a severe arch and requires that the position be held while the head moves independently. Therefore, look to evenly distribute the extension throughout the spine rather than allowing it to be focused in the highly mobile L5/S1 junction.

Single Leg Kick

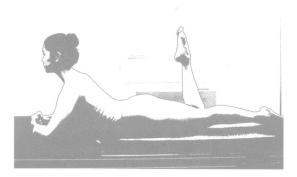

Shoulder Bridge

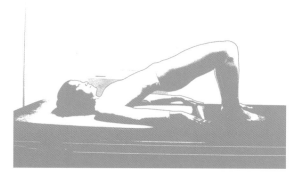

Neck Roll

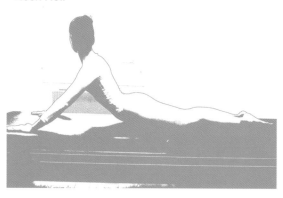

7

FORWARD LUNGE

and Foot/Ankle Instability

This exercise requires steady ankle alignment and can therefore reveal or exacerbate any weaknesses in the joint.

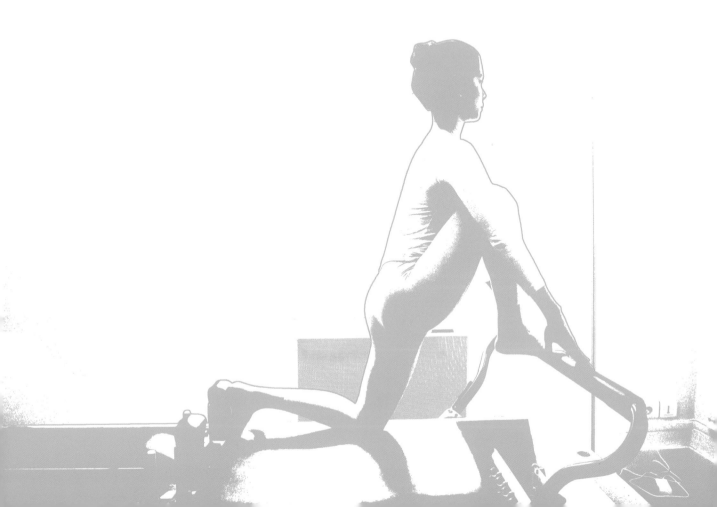

Principles of the Exercise

Starting Position

Forward Lunge is a version of a front split that calls for very specific placement of the feet—one on the carriage against the shoulder rest, the other with the toes on the bar and the heel raised. One knee is on the carriage, and the knee closer to the bar is free. The hands are placed symmetrically on either side of the trunk to help maintain balance.

Note that the feet are in two different positions: The foot on the carriage is in *dorsiflexion,* with the toes turned toward the shin. The foot on the bar, at least at the beginning of the exercise, is in *plantar flexion,* which we call "pointed."

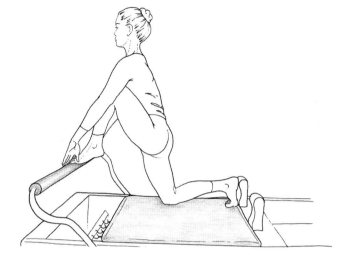

The Movement

Both knees start to straighten to press the carriage out. The instep of the foot on the bar is forced into a more extreme point, and the foot on the carriage goes into more extreme extension. This pattern is reversed on the return.

Throughout this exercise, we try to stabilize the pelvis and keep it from turning. The two feet move differently. The back foot moves from a flexed to a more pointed position (in that the heel pulls away from the shoulder rest). The front foot goes from a pointed to a less pointed position.

Observations

In the course of this exercise, the foot on the bar often turns and changes shape. Why?

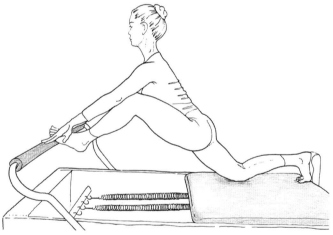

When we place the foot in a point on the bar, it simultaneously:

✦ twists on itself so that the sole is turned inward (and not toward the floor); and
✦ tends to move to the lateral side, which brings the heel more toward the little toe.

This movement occurs at the ankle and involves several other joints of the foot as well.

Anatomical Landmarks

The Ankle: A Structure Composed of Two Joints

The upper portion of the ankle joint is itself composed of two superimposed joints—the ends of the two bones of the lower leg, the tibia and the fibula. The ankle can thus be more precisely recognized as the tibia-fibula-talus.

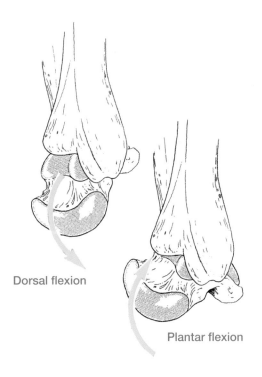

Dorsal flexion

Plantar flexion

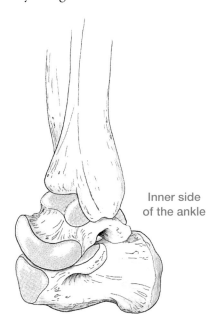

Inner side
of the ankle

The ends of the tibia and the fibula fit snugly together like a monkey wrench over the upper part of the talus, which resembles the top of a pulley wheel. The two "fingers" of the wrench correspond to the malleoli. This joint allows only for front and back movement:

✦ to the front, dorsal flexion (dorsiflexion)
✦ to the back, plantar flexion

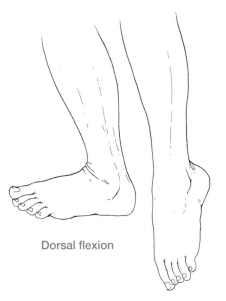

Dorsal flexion

Plantar flexion

The ankle bones are generally stable, but there is some room for movement in certain positions. In plantar flexion, for instance, we can see that the posterior part of the "pulley," which is narrower than the front, is in the monkey wrench. Because it's narrower, it fits less snugly, and there is therefore room for tiny lateral and rotational movements. Even though the movement is minimal, it means that the ankle is less stable in this position—at least when we look exclusively at the bones.

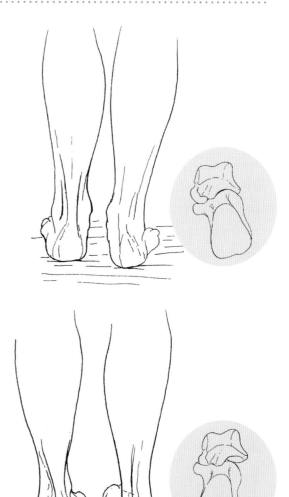

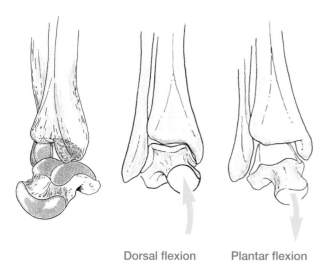

Dorsal flexion   Plantar flexion

The Lower Heel: Talus-Calcaneus

Two surfaces on the underside of the talus articulate with two corresponding surfaces on the top of the calcaneum. This area of articulation (illustrated at right) allows for a greater diversity of movement, but with less range of motion than at the ankle. Lateral movement is dominant here.

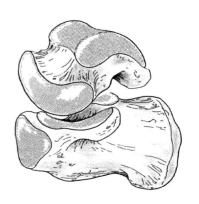

The Instep:
The Midtarsal and
Tarsometatarsal Joints

At the front of the ankle is the instep, which joins two articular lines, each one involving several bones. The Forward Lunge exposes the instep of the foot on the bar.

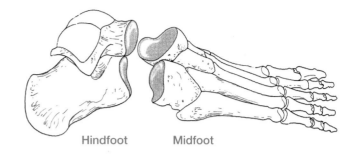

Hindfoot   Midfoot

————————————————

Midtarsal joint

The Tarsometatarsal
(the Joint at the Front of the Instep)
The tarsometatarsal joint unites the bones of the midfoot with the five metatarsals. It allows for the same movement as the midtarsal joint, although with less mobility.

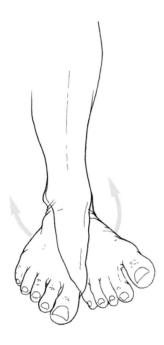

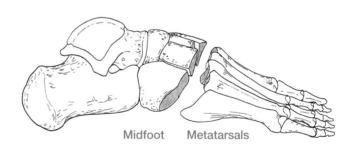

Midfoot   Metatarsals

————————————————

Tarsometatarsal joint

The Midtarsal
(the Joint Behind the Instep)
The midtarsal unites the calcaneum and the talus with the two bones situated more anteriorly. It is the first joint of the foot that is on a vertical plane.

The midtarsal joint can make the same types of movement as those made by the subtalar joint. It permits the hindfoot to adapt to the midfoot, especially when they are bearing weight, as when the foot is on the bar.

These multiple joints increase the foot's movement possibilities, but they can make alignment more complicated. Therefore, ankle support and alignment most often require coordination of the surrounding muscles.

Consequences

Plantar Flexion Encourages Inversion

When movements of the ankle and foot employ all of the joints described above, two results predominate: inversion and eversion. When the ankle goes into plantar flexion, inversion tends to occur. Inversion combines three movements. The ankle goes into plantar flexion, while the joints below and in front of the ankle tend to:

+ supinate (meaning that the internal edge of the foot lifts, while the external edge drops); and
+ adduct (the instep turns toward the midline of the body).

Why this combination? Generally speaking, inversion is a result of both the shape of the articulating surfaces and the predominant muscular action: most of the muscles that cause plantar flexion are also supinators.

In effect, an unstable talus is guided by the action of the dominant muscles, which in this case are supinators. In Forward Lunge, the foot that is held in plantar flexion will tend not to stay aligned, but to move into inversion.

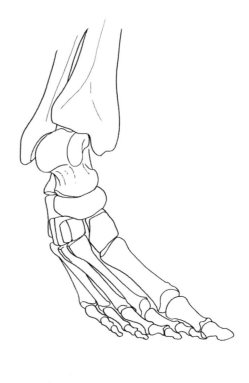

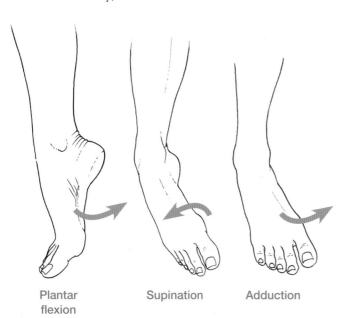

Plantar   Supination   Adduction
flexion

The Consequences of Inversion

Inversion moves the talus and the calcaneum away from the lateral malleolus. When this happens, the ligaments at the outside of the ankle are put under tension.

The Ankle and Its Outer Ligaments

The lateral malleolus has a "V" shape: its two edges meet in a point. It has ligaments that connect it both to the talus and to the calcaneum.

+ In the front, a ligament runs from the anterior edge to the talus (1).
+ At the bottom, a ligament runs from the point to the calcaneum (2).
+ In the back, a ligament runs from the posterior edge to the talus (3).

These three ligaments provide stability for the ankle. They are put under tension during inversion.

Inversion Particularly Stretches the Anterior Ligament

Among the three ligaments, the one that is stretched the most in inversion is the anterior ligament. This is the ligament that is most often overstretched and injured when the ankle is twisted.

In Forward Lunge, the foot tends to go into a position where the ankle is in torsion. Even if this doesn't directly cause a twisted ankle, it might predispose you to one.

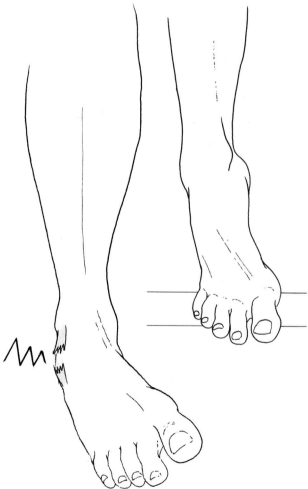

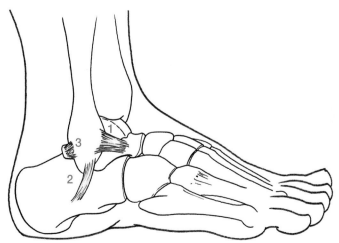

Solutions and Prevention

How to Stabilize the Foot

The way to prevent ankle strain is to stabilize the foot during Forward Lunge and other similar exercises.

1. Define Optimal Leg Alignment from the Hip to the Knee

This can be done standing on the mat, with the legs parallel and about hip width apart.

✦ Internally rotate the femurs and note how the knees turn inward toward each other. The tibias will follow the same pattern and bring the taluses with them.

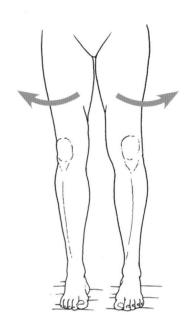

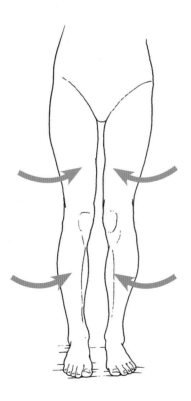

✦ Do the opposite and turn the hips into external rotation (by contracting the glutes, for example). This time the kneecaps will turn outward. The tibias, which are pulled into external rotation, will bring the taluses into supination.

✦ You can find a balance between the two positions. The legs will be just slightly more externally rotated, and this will allow the kneecaps to face forward and avoid supination or pronation of the feet.*

---

*For more information on this exercise, see Blandine Calais-Germain's *Anatomy of Movement*.

2. The Plié

To coordinate the entire lower extremity, one of the best exercises is still the plié.

Start in the same position as in the previous exercise, standing on the mat with the legs parallel and about hip width apart. While the plié actually requires alignment of the entire body, here we will focus on hip-knee-foot alignment.*

+ Bring the legs together so that the big toes, the medial malleoli, and the knees touch. Bend the knees, keeping the heels on the mat and the three points (toes, malleoli, and knees) touching.

+ Once you have mastered this step, separate the legs to hip width apart and go into a plié, keeping the ankles in the same position as when the legs were touching.

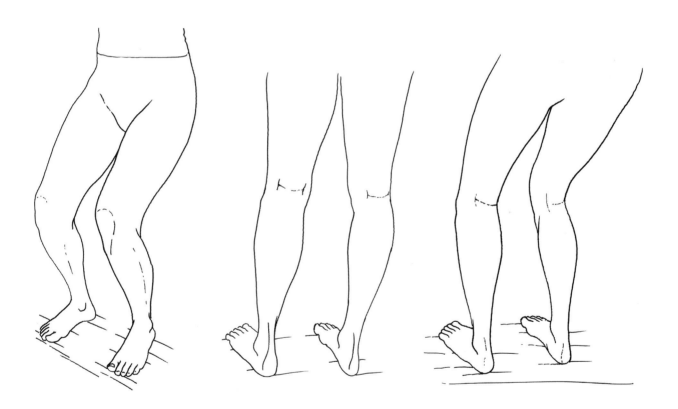

*For more information on this exercise, see Blandine Calais-Germain's *Anatomy of Movement*.

3. Come into Demi-Point

Stand with the legs and feet together. Come up into a demi-point—putting your weight on the metatarsals. Initially, while keeping the legs together, we try to keep the malleoli in contact (1). If they separate (2), this is because the feet are starting to go into inversion.

Next, separate the legs. While maintaining the same knee-ankle-foot alignment, come up onto the metatarsals and then lower the heels (3). This is the time to discover whether your heels drop to the outside (supinate) when you raise them. If so, practice raising them without supinating.

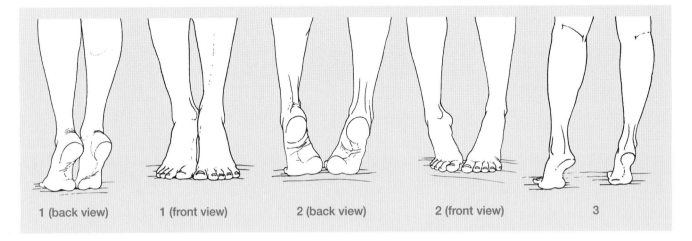

1 (back view)   1 (front view)   2 (back view)   2 (front view)   3

4. Prevent Supination

Supination of the foot—and thereby inversion—can also be caused by the knee dropping outward (1). At first, we try to keep the knee aligned with the hip and foot. We can even try dropping it slightly inward (2).

Later, if we allow the knee to drop slightly outward (via abduction and external rotation of the hip), we will specifically be able to avoid letting the foot rock to the outer limit of its area of contact (3).

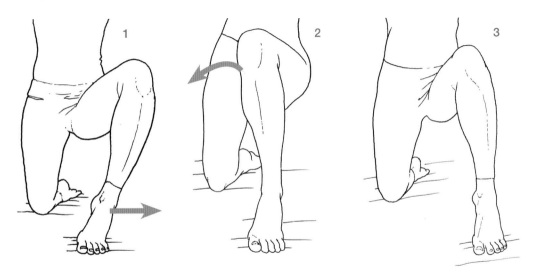

Other Exercises That Encourage Ankle Instability

Reformer Exercises

All of the exercises that put pressure on the foot will be challenging to the ankle. Here, we focus on those that involve plantar flexion.

Footwork

In this series, there are variations such as Tendon Stretch and Running where the toes are on the bar and there is a tendency to fall to the outside of the foot.

Stomach Massage

In this series, we see the same inversion of the foot when the toes are on the bar in the basic exercise and the variations.

Footwork (Tendon Stretch)

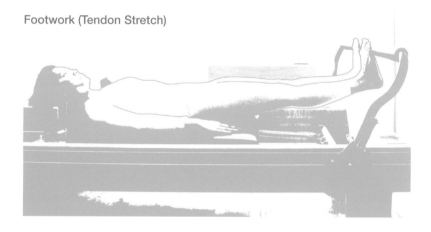

Footwork (Running)

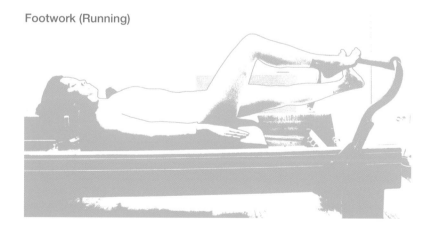

Long Stretch, Up Stretch, Arabesque, Front Split

In these four exercises, there is a strong tendency to plantar inversion since both feet are in demi-point.

Semi-circle

This position of extreme plantar flexion encourages the foot to drop outward.

Long Stretch

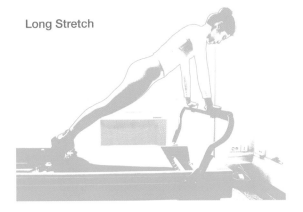

Up Stretch

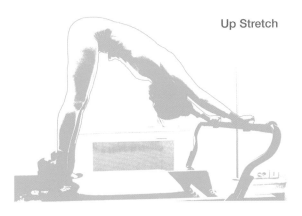

Front Split

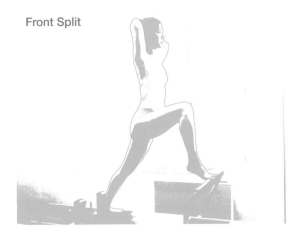

Semi-circle

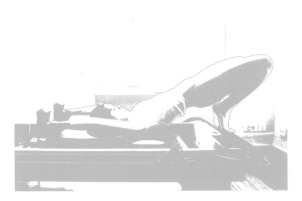

Mat Exercises

There are not many mat exercises that call for the weight of the body to be supported on the feet. However, both the Push-up series and Leg Pull Front can create inversion of the ankles.

Push-up Series and Leg Pull Front

These two exercises that involve putting weight on the hands and the feet can cause inversion problems. In both cases, the solution is to focus the weight on the axis of the foot that passes through the second toe. This helps prevent the foot from turning to the outside.

Push-up Series

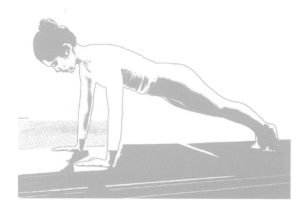

Leg Pull Front

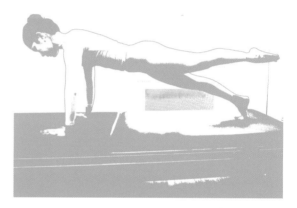

8

SIDE SIT-UPS (SHORT BOX)

and the Vertebral Ligaments

This exercise is done with the box on the carriage of the Reformer. It specifically involves lateral inclination and back torsion of the thoracic and lumbar spine.

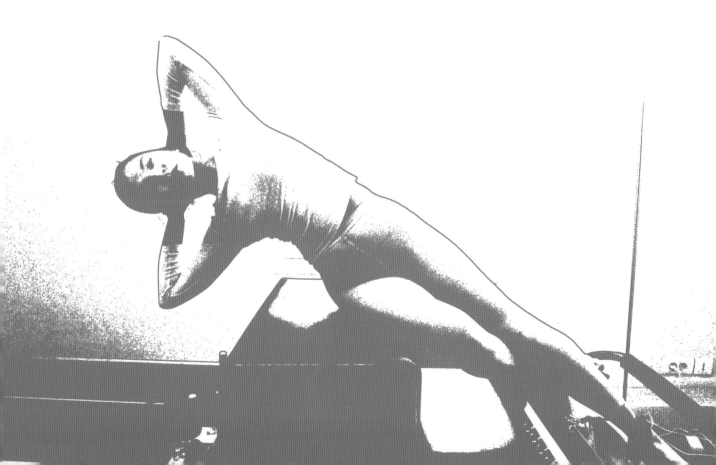

Principles of the Exercise

Starting Position

Start by sitting on the box on the left hip. Extend the right leg and place it under the strap. The left leg is bent and the ankle is wrapped around the right calf.

The hands are placed one on top of the other at the base of the neck.

The Movement

In this exercise, the carriage doesn't move. It's the height of the box that we use, rather than the spring resistance.

✦ First, we start in a vertical position, and then extend the trunk out so that it is on the same line as the leg that is under the strap.

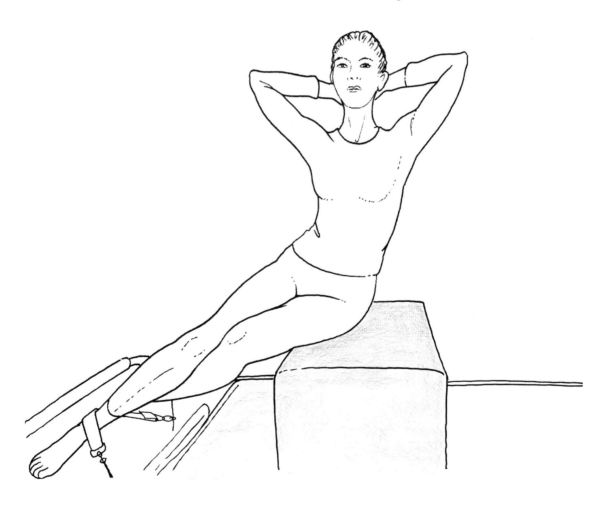

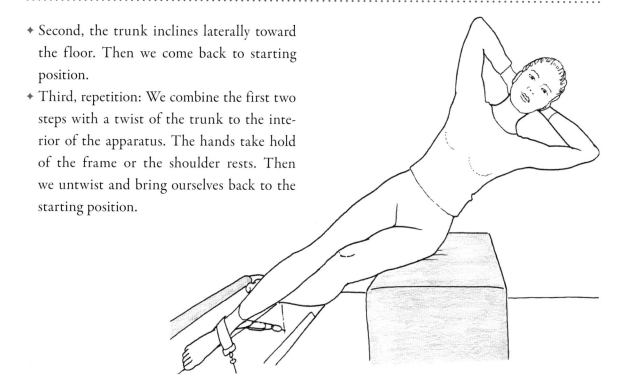

✦ Second, the trunk inclines laterally toward the floor. Then we come back to starting position.

✦ Third, repetition: We combine the first two steps with a twist of the trunk to the interior of the apparatus. The hands take hold of the frame or the shoulder rests. Then we untwist and bring ourselves back to the starting position.

Observations

The Side Sit-ups exercise is composed of two movements in sequence: inclination and torsion, or rotation. We tend to mix and combine these two movements when doing several repetitions, which can strain the joints of the spinal column. This is especially true when the range of motion is extreme, and when we don't know how to properly initiate rotation. Why?

We need to start by observing the two movements separately.

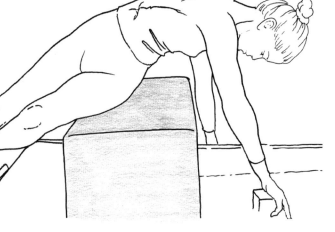

Anatomical Landmarks

Inclination

Inclination curves the spine laterally, giving the trunk a concave side and a convex side. At each level of the curve, there are consequences for all of the anatomical elements involved.

On the *concave* side:

+ The intervertebral disk is squeezed.
+ The lateral ligaments are compressed.
+ The muscles are compressed.

The lateral ligaments run from one transverse apophysis (a lateral projection of the vertebrae) to the next.

On the *convex* side:

+ The intervertebral disk is stretched.
+ The nucleus tends to move to this side.
+ The intertransverse ligaments are put under tension.
+ The muscles are put under tension.

The more pronounced the curve, the more profound the effects, and the more moderate the curve, the less profound these effects will be.

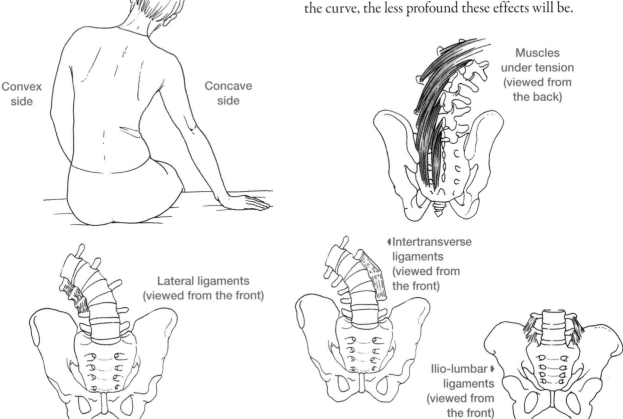

Convex side

Concave side

Muscles under tension (viewed from the back)

Lateral ligaments (viewed from the front)

◀Intertransverse ligaments (viewed from the front)

Ilio-lumbar ▶ ligaments (viewed from the front)

*Ligament Irregularities
during Inclination*

On the lowest vertebrae, the lateral ligaments are the ilio-lumbar ligaments. Their transverse apophyses are anchored to the iliac crests. These very powerful ligaments are designed to restrict lateral inclination. Extreme lateral inclination at this level can damage these ligaments, which like all ligaments do not have much give.

Rotation (Torsion)

Rotation is influenced by the shape of the articular aphophyses that meet at each level of the spine. These apophyses form the facet joints at the back of the vertebrae.

The Lumbar Region Does Not Rotate

At the level of the lumbar spine, the superior articulating surfaces are shaped like hollow cylinders. The inferior articulating surfaces are like full cylinders. In a stack of two vertebrae, these surfaces push against each other bit by bit, and the hollow cylinders tend to push the full cylinders laterally (1).

This arrangement permits flexion, extension, and lateral inclination but almost totally impedes any one lumbar vertebra from rotating on top of or under another.

If we try to force rotation in this area, the articular surfaces separate on the side of the rotation, placing the ligaments and capsules under tension. Opposite the side of rotation, the articular surfaces are put under pressure, resulting in compression of the cartilage.

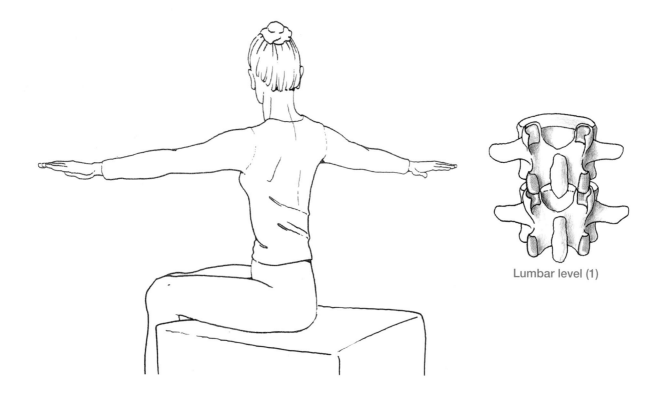

Lumbar level (1)

Rotation Is Possible in the Thoracic Spine

The four surfaces of the thoracic articular apophyses are flat. These apophyseal planes form part of the circle whose center is the body of the vertebra. This is a feature that encourages rotation (2).

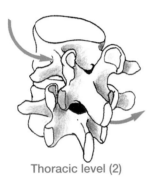

Thoracic level (2)

Mobility Is Not the Same at All Levels of the Thoracic Spine

The presence of the thoracic rib cage notably reduces the amplitude of rotation, especially in the upper ribs (1–7), which are directly connected to the sternum. The lower ribs are not as restricted, however, and their vertebrae rotate more easily. The most mobile vertebrae are on either side of the T11/T12 junction.

If we strongly augment the range of rotation at the thoracic level, the articulating surfaces separate and this puts their capsules and ligaments under tension.

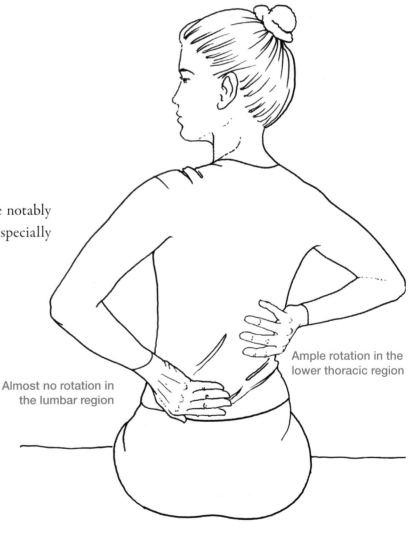

Almost no rotation in the lumbar region

Ample rotation in the lower thoracic region

Consequences

The "Overhang"

When we look at lateral inclination (combined with rotation) in Side Sit-ups, we see that the spine is not vertical in line with gravity; rather, the upper part of the spine (the head) is displaced laterally relative to the lower spine (the pelvis). This creates an overhang.

The effect of this overhang on the lower vertebrae, which support the weight of the upper body, is that the weight of the upper body is multiplied by the amount of displacement. The load is therefore augmented on all of the lower vertebrae. The greater the amplitude of displacement, the greater the load on the lower vertebrae.

Overhang Increases the Effects of Inclination

As we discussed on page 97, inclination creates tension and compression in the spine.

✦ On the concave side of the curve, the compression of the disks is augmented.
✦ On the convex side of the curve, the disks and ligaments are put under more tension.

Overhang Also Multiplies the Effects of Rotation

Rotation itself can also increase the overhang.

✦ Pressure is increased on the surfaces of the lumbar articular apophyses.

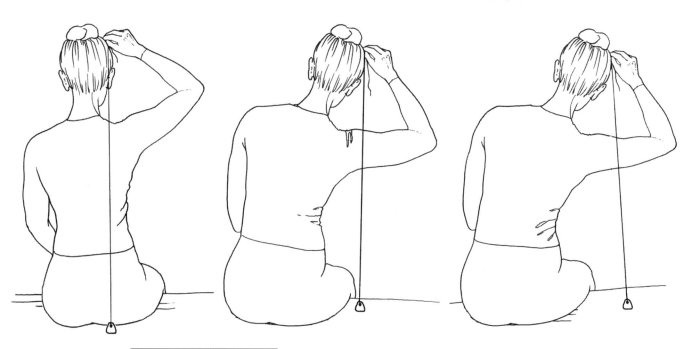

Inclination causes the head and upper spine to "hang over" the lower spine.

✦ The capsules and ligaments of the thoracic articular apophyses are put under more tension as well.

Summary of the Effects of Side Sit-ups

When Side Sit-ups are performed at their maximum range of motion, the spine can be adversely affected in many ways and in several different areas at once.

Effects of Inclination

When the spine is inclined during Side Sit-ups, the following changes can be observed:

✦ The disks are pinched and compressed dramatically on the concave side (1) and forcefully stretched on the convex side. Again we see the same sort of risks that we saw with the yo-yo effect in chapter 1.
✦ The nucleus tends to migrate to the convex side. Here, we see the same risk of disk herniation that we saw in chapter 3.
✦ The ligaments are forcefully stretched on the convex side. The intertransverse ligaments (2) and ilio-lumbar ligaments (3) can be stretched beyond their limit. This can cause pain and ligament distention and can also create intervertebral instability, wherein the ligaments lose their ability to provide support and leave the spine quite fragile.

Effects of Rotation/Torsion

When the spine is rotated to its maximum point, the following changes can occur:

✦ On the concave side, the weight on the surfaces of the lumbar articular apophyses is increased. This excess pressure can damage the articular cartilage.
✦ Under tension, the capsules and ligaments of the lumbar articular apophyses can get sore.

Combining Inclination and Rotation

When inclination and rotation are combined, the spine is quite vulnerable to injury.

The muscles of the convex side are stretched (4), yet they are also contracted. While this contraction is limited, it is active, and it can cause all of the problems mentioned above.

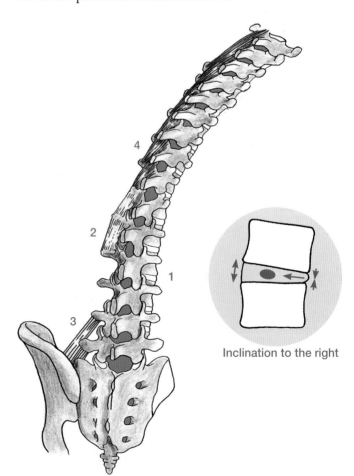

Inclination to the right

Solutions and Prevention

How to Avoid the Overhang in Lateral Inclination

Because the spine is so vulnerable during Side Sit-ups, it is important to find ways of avoiding the phenomenon of "overhang."

1. Discover How Lateral Inclination Should Feel in a "Non-loaded" Position

Before you try to find your range of lateral movement in the exercise, it's interesting to explore an appropriate range of motion on the mat. Here, the effects of the gravity load are eliminated.

To laterally incline to the right:

+ Bring your left arm above your head while keeping it as close to the floor as possible, then tip the trunk to the right.
+ Augment the movement by bringing the right hand toward the right heel as if you were trying to get them to meet. Then come back to the starting position.

Before moving to the other side, it's interesting to repeat the movement several times on one side so the you don't confuse the two feelings. Chances are the range will be different

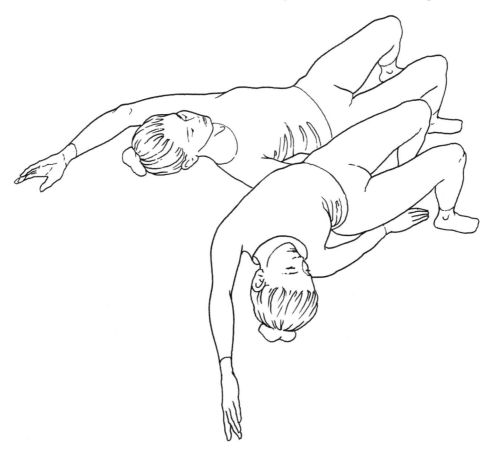

on the two sides. Feel your convex (left) side as it stretches all the way out to the sides of the waist and the ribs, as well as the sensation of the vertebrae opening.

2. Control the Amplitude of the Movement

Repeat the exercise in a non-loaded position. This time, throughout the movement, try not to close the right (concave) side of the curve; instead, imagine that you're lengthening it. This recruits the muscles on the convex side—the muscles on the side of the larger curve—which will stabilize the spine in a less extreme position.

This effort employs the deep muscles of the spine as well as the superficial trunk muscles, and even the obliques. It's helpful to feel the muscles that brake the movement. Their sensations are often confused with those of a stretch, even though these are different actions.

3. Avoid Lumbar Rotation by Practicing Thoracic Rotation

When rotating the spine, we can keep the lumbar spine relatively stable. The best way to do this is to practice thoracic rotation.

This can be done while seated on the box, where the range of the pelvis is the greatest and the hamstrings are relaxed.

+ Put your hands on your ribs and keep your pelvis facing the bar. When you initiate the movement, start the rotation with the ribs, and keep the pelvis stable.
+ Try to rotate evenly throughout the spine and avoid favoring the T11/T12 junction. In other words, try to make the rotation as high as possible. Come back to center, and change sides.

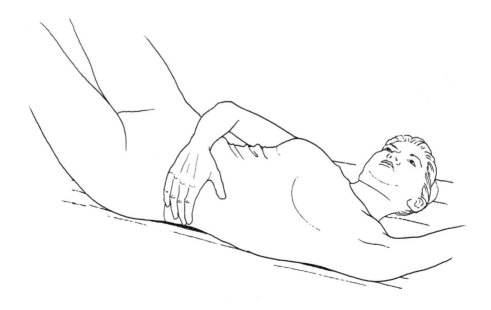

4. Modify the Exercise

Before attempting the full Side Sit-up, break it down into two separate sequences:

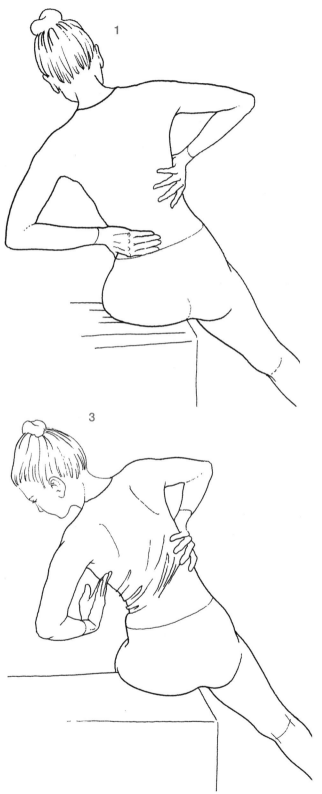

+ Work on the head-heel alignment before going into lateral inclination (1).
+ Start the torsion from this aligned position and not from an inclined position (2). This will still create an overhang, but since the spine isn't curved, the spinal structures will be less stressed.
+ Ensure that the pelvis hasn't internally rotated when thoracic rotation is initiated.
+ Finally, start the inclination mainly from the thoracic spine (where we see the folds in the clothing in the illustration) (3).

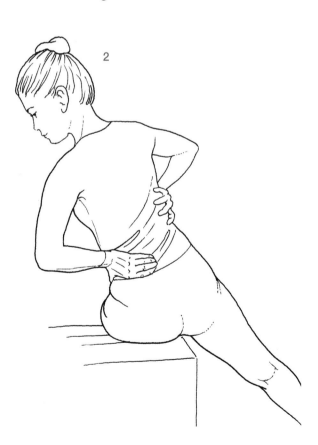

Other Exercises That Carry Similar Risks for the Spine

Reformer Exercises

The following exercises involve lateral rotation or inclination, or both.

Stomach Massage Twist

The Twist is a variation on the basic Stomach Massage. Rotation is added to a position that already stretches the hamstrings and flexes the lower back. In this position, the rotation shouldn't be made by the arms, which are stretched out—one to the front and one to the back. That is to say, torsion needs to be made from the ribs and not by momentum of the upper extremities.

It's best not to attempt this version of the series until the hamstrings are flexible enough so that you can perform it without flexing the lower back.

Short Box Side-to-Side

An exercise based on lateral inclination, this one is done on the box with the arms vertical while you hold a bar in your hands. The bar can help you keep the movement in the frontal plane and control the range of the lateral curve.

Short Box Twist with Reach

The starting position for this variation is the same as for the preceding one: seated on the box, arms vertical, bar in hands. Then we rotate the torso and dip the trunk to the back while aligning it with the legs. This position is loaded, but the disks are aligned. To perform this exercise correctly, the initial torsion needs to be made at the level of the ribs and not lower.

This should bring to mind the Twist, which is a progression of the Snake, and holds the same risks as the exercises presented above.

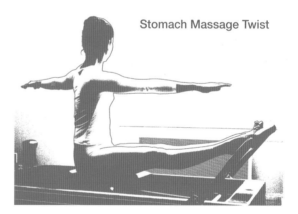

Stomach Massage Twist

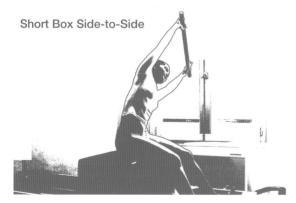

Short Box Side-to-Side

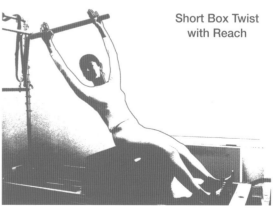

Short Box Twist
with Reach

Mat Exercises

The following mat exercises can also injure the vertebral ligaments.

Crisscross

This is a sort of scissoring/crossing movement done on the mat. The upper torso turns toward the opposite knee, which is bent and moves toward the elbow. The particular position of this abdominal exercise is a good way to feel where the rotation should be made. Rotation should not move to the lumbar area, and the lower back should not move.

Crisscross

Saw

Sit on the floor, with your legs separated and arms open to the sides. This exercise combines torsion, back flexion, and a stretch of the lumbar area. Instead of accentuating lumbar flexion, it's preferable to control rotation (accentuating torsion of the back) before attempting to glide the opposite hand toward the foot. It's preferable at this stage to limit the flexion to the level of the ribs.

Saw

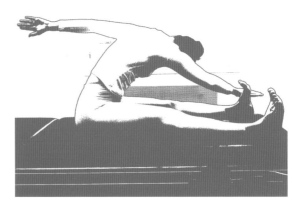

Mermaid Stretch

A variation of lateral inclination with the knees bent to the side. We see here, as in other exercises of this nature, that it is key to keep the waist long to keep the lateral inclination in a safe range.

Mermaid Stretch

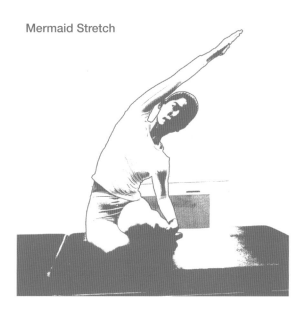

Spine Twist

This is a version of the Saw without flexion of the trunk. The starting position is the same except that the legs are together instead of separated, and we make two twists to each side. Here too, avoid using the impetus of the arms to force the rotation. It's the arms that follow the movement of the ribs and not vice versa.

Spine Twist

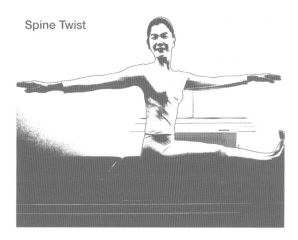

SUMMARY CHART

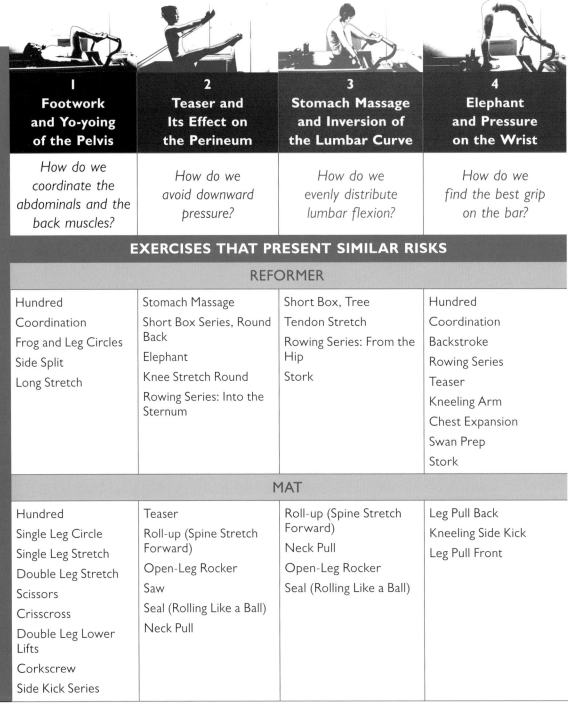

1 **Footwork and Yo-yoing of the Pelvis**	2 **Teaser and Its Effect on the Perineum**	3 **Stomach Massage and Inversion of the Lumbar Curve**	4 **Elephant and Pressure on the Wrist**
How do we coordinate the abdominals and the back muscles?	*How do we avoid downward pressure?*	*How do we evenly distribute lumbar flexion?*	*How do we find the best grip on the bar?*
EXERCISES THAT PRESENT SIMILAR RISKS			
REFORMER			
Hundred Coordination Frog and Leg Circles Side Split Long Stretch	Stomach Massage Short Box Series, Round Back Elephant Knee Stretch Round Rowing Series: Into the Sternum	Short Box, Tree Tendon Stretch Rowing Series: From the Hip Stork	Hundred Coordination Backstroke Rowing Series Teaser Kneeling Arm Chest Expansion Swan Prep Stork
MAT			
Hundred Single Leg Circle Single Leg Stretch Double Leg Stretch Scissors Crisscross Double Leg Lower Lifts Corkscrew Side Kick Series	Teaser Roll-up (Spine Stretch Forward) Open-Leg Rocker Saw Seal (Rolling Like a Ball) Neck Pull	Roll-up (Spine Stretch Forward) Neck Pull Open-Leg Rocker Seal (Rolling Like a Ball)	Leg Pull Back Kneeling Side Kick Leg Pull Front

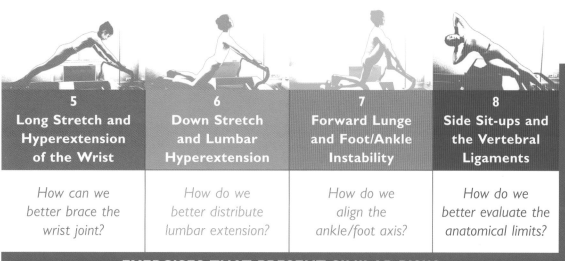

5 **Long Stretch and Hyperextension of the Wrist**	6 **Down Stretch and Lumbar Hyperextension**	7 **Forward Lunge and Foot/Ankle Instability**	8 **Side Sit-ups and the Vertebral Ligaments**
How can we better brace the wrist joint?	*How do we better distribute lumbar extension?*	*How do we align the ankle/foot axis?*	*How do we better evaluate the anatomical limits?*
EXERCISES THAT PRESENT SIMILAR RISKS			
REFORMER			
Kneeling Arm Series Knees Off Tendon Stretch	Swan Prep Hamstring Curls Snake Knee Stretch (Arched)	Footwork Stomach Massage Long Stretch Up Stretch Arabesque Front Split Semi-circle	Stomach Massage Twist Short Box: ✦ Side-to-Side ✦ Twist with Reach
MAT			
Leg Pull Front Kneeling Side Kick Mermaid Stretch Leg Pull Back	Swimming Single Leg Kick Double Leg Kick Shoulder Bridge Neck Roll	Push-up Series Leg Pull Front	Crisscross Saw Mermaid Stretch Spine Twist

FURTHER READING

Books by Blandine Calais-Germain

Anatomy of Breathing. Seattle: Eastland Press, 2006.

Anatomy of Movement. Rev. ed. Seattle: Eastland Press, 2007.

Anatomy of Movement: Exercises (with Andrée Lamotte). Seattle: Eastland Press, 2008.

The Female Pelvis: Anatomy & Exercises. Seattle: Eastland Press, 2003.

No-Risk Abs: A Safe Workout Program for Core Strength. Rochester, Vt.: Healing Arts Press, 2011.

Preparing for a Gentle Birth: The Pelvis in Pregnancy. Rochester, Vt.: Healing Arts Press, 2011.

Recommended Pilates Reading

Curtis-Oakes, Martine. *Perfect Pilates: L'art de modeler son corps.* Paris: Editions Vigot, 2005.

Recommended Anatomy Books

Basmajiann, John V. *Primary Anatomy.* Champaign, Ill.: Stipes Publishing, 1998.

Bouchet, Alain, and Jacques Cuilleret. *Anatomie topographique, descriptive et fonctionnelle.* Paris: Simep/Masson, 1991.

Brizon, Jacques, and Jean Castaing. *Les feuillets d'anatomie.* Paris: Editions Maloine, 1996.

Kapandji, Ibrahim Adalbert. *The Physiology of the Joints.* 3 vols. 6th ed. London: Churchill Livingstone, 2007 and 2008.

Platzer, Werner. *Color Atlas of Human Anatomy: Locomotor System*. 6th ed. New York: Thieme, 2009.

Vandervael, Franz. *Analyse des mouvements du corps humain*. Paris: Editions Maloine, 1958.

Vigué-Martin. *Atlas of the Human Body*. Surrey, UK: Rebo International BV, 2005.

INDEX

Books of Related Interest

No-Risk Abs
A Safe Workout Program for Core Strength
by Blandine Calais-Germain

Weight-Resistance Yoga
Practicing Embodied Spirituality
by Max Popov

The New Rules of Posture
How to Sit, Stand, and Move in the Modern World
by Mary Bond

Pilates on the Ball
A Comprehensive Book and DVD Workout
by Colleen Craig

The Five Tibetans
Five Dynamic Exercises for Health, Energy, and Personal Power
by Christopher S. Kilham

The Heart of Yoga
Developing a Personal Practice
by T. K. V. Desikachar

Bioharmonic Self-Massage
How to Harmonize Your Mental, Emotional, and Physical Energies
by Yves Bligny

Primal Body, Primal Mind
Beyond the Paleo Diet for Total Health and a Longer Life
by Nora T. Gedgaudas, CNS, CNT

INNER TRADITIONS • BEAR & COMPANY
P.O. Box 388
Rochester, VT 05767
1-800-246-8648
www.InnerTraditions.com

Or contact your local bookseller